# WHAT THE EX|

"Dr. McKenna's work provides the ~~~~~~~~~~~~~~~~ | we
have been able to illustrate the saf ~~~~~~~~~~~~~~ : in his
sleep lab has led us to understand why mothers and infants do what they
do, and his sheer exuberance, energy, and enthusiasm has made this such an
enjoyable lesson along the way."

> —Peter S. Blair, Ph.D., Professor of Epidemiology and Statistics, Centre for
> Academic Child Health, Bristol Medical School, University of Bristol

"This is a very detailed and comprehensive narrative about everything to do
with cosleeping, through the unique lens of a dedicated academic who has
devoted most of his professional career to this topic. Parents who are keen to
understand the historical controversies around cosleeping, and to know more
about how SIDS epidemiology and sleep science are conducted, will find
much to think about here."

> —Helen Ball, Ph.D., M.A., B.Sc., Professor of Anthropology, Durham
> University, Director of the Durham Infancy & Sleep Centre, Co-Director of
> the Baby Sleep Information Source

"Once you have read James McKenna's satisfying and intuitive book, you will
finally get a good night's sleep: He will free you of worrying about 'creating
bad sleep habits' and help you stop feeling unsure about breastfeeding your
baby to sleep."

> —Jack Newman, M.D., F.R.C.P.C., I.B.C.L.C., and Andrea Polokova, M.A.,
> M.Ed., co-authors of *Breastfeeding: Empowering Parents*

"Dr. McKenna seamlessly integrates his own scientific research and that of
others with history, anthropological concepts, and maternal instinct, while
demonstrating how the Western cultural bias of independent sleep actually
increases the risk of SIDS and poor long-term adjustment."

> —Nancy E. Wight, M.D., I.B.C.L.C., F.A.B.M., F.A.A.P., Neonatologist,
> Medical Director for Sharp HealthCare Lactation Services

"[Cosleeping] is not for everyone, but Dr. McKenna has brought it into
focus as a good choice for many parents, and has rightly questioned official
attempts to suppress it based on rare and avoidable events. In this easy-to-
read, thoroughly informed book, parents will find what they need to know to
cosleep safely. An important contribution to the literature on baby care, and
especially to the attachment parenting movement."

> —Melvin Konner, M.D., Ph.D., Samuel Candler Dobbs Professor of
> Anthropology and of Neuroscience & Behavioral Biology, Emory
> University, author of *The Evolution of Childhood*

"A detailed explanation of what cosleeping is, what it implies for the health of
mother and baby, and how to practice it safely. An indispensable reading for
all parents who want to decide in a conscious and well-informed way where
and how their baby should sleep...."

> —María Berrozpe Martínez, Ph.D., author of *¡Dulces Sueños!* (*Sweet Sleep!*),
> co-author of *Una Nueva Maternidad* (*A New Motherhood*), instructor for La
> Leche League International

"Dr. McKenna will show you your options and teach you how to reduce the risk of infant death and prolong breastfeeding. This book is a must-read for every new parent."

—Kathleen Kendall-Tackett, Ph.D., I.B.C.L.C., F.A.P.A., co-author of *Breastfeeding Made Simple* and *The Science of Mother-Infant Sleep*

"I have been a pediatrician for over 40 years. There has never been an occurrence of SIDS in my practice. I might be good... but I'm not that good. Virtually every single family in my practice safely cosleeps. They all are breastsleeping families."

—Jay Gordon, M.D., Fellow of the American Academy of Pediatrics, co-author of *Good Nights: The Happy Parents' Guide to the Family Bed (and a Peaceful Night's Sleep!)*

"As the father of four sons and as a practicing pediatrician, developmental physiologist, and epidemiologist, I can strongly support the ideas presented by Dr. McKenna in this debunking of much of the arrogant, ill-informed, and misleading advice that has in the past been given to parents by professionals who should have known better. I wholeheartedly commend this book to parents and to healthcare professionals."

—Peter J. Fleming, C.B.E., F.R.S.A., Ph.D., M.B.Ch.B., F.R.C.P. (Canada, London), F.R.C.P.C.H., Professor of Infant Health and Developmental Physiology, Consultant Paediatrician, Centre for Academic Child Health, Population Health Sciences, Bristol Medical School, University of Bristol

"Dr. McKenna is the world's leading expert on cosleeping, its evolutionary story, and its importance to parents. In his new book, he shares that knowledge with parents in our society. I strongly recommend it to new parents."

—Robert A. LeVine, Ph.D., Professor Emeritus of Education and Human Development, Harvard University

"Families who are confused, scared, and frustrated by our current black and white messaging seek information to understand why, if bedsharing feels so instinctually safe, they should avoid it. This book is a greatly-needed resource that provides evidence for families to make educated decisions when trying to balance their instincts about breastsleeping and bedsharing with the advice given to them by American society."

—Anne Eglash M.D., I.B.C.L.C., F.A.B.M., Director of Lactation Services, University of Wisconsin School of Medicine and Public Health, Founder and President of The Institute for the Advancement of Breastfeeding and Lactation Education (IABLE)

"Professor McKenna is not afraid to take a stand on this controversial issue, presenting the view that bedsharing in the absence of hazardous circumstances can bring many benefits to infants and families; that it is the way infants sleep, not where they sleep, that is important. This review of the subject is likely of benefit to anyone considering bedsharing."

—Sally Baddock, B.Sc., Dip. Tchng., Ph.D., Professor, School of Midwifery, Otago Polytechnic, New Zealand

"To cosleep or not to cosleep? That's the question vexing so many new parents. From over 20 years of groundbreaking research in his Mother-Baby Behavioral Sleep Lab, biological anthropologist James McKenna knows more than anyone about the risks and benefits of cosleeping. If you're looking for a sound, scientific basis for deciding about whether, when, where, how, and why to cosleep safely with your baby, look no farther—this book will tell you all you need to know."

>—Alma Gottlieb, Ph.D., Professor of Anthropology, University of Illinois, Urbana-Champaign, co-author of *A World of Babies: Imagined Childcare Guides for Eight Societies*

"Brilliant! Dr. McKenna, a research scientist who has spent much of his academic career studying bedsharing and its relationship to maternal and child health, has provided us with a vital resource to all who care about infants, parenting issues, public health issues—both mental and physical— and our society in general. It is with great pride that I recommend this book to the breastfeeding world and the world at large."

>—Chele Marmet, B.S., M.A., F.I.L.C.A., pioneer of the lactation consultant profession

"Dr. McKenna presents the benefits and risks of shared sleeping with babies and proposes strategies to create safer shared sleeping environments that support a risk minimization approach, which is evidence-based and practical for families to tailor to their individual needs and circumstances."

>—Jeanine Young, F.A.C.N., Ph.D., R.G.N., Registered Midwife, Professor, University of the Sunshine Coast, member of the Red Nose National Scientific Advisory Group

"With overwhelming evidence and unparalleled heart, the brilliant Professor McKenna shreds the conventional misguidance to reclaim the mammal universal of safe cosleeping for better health and well-being of mothers and babies."

>—Katie Hinde, Ph.D., Associate Professor, Center for Evolution and Medicine, Arizona State University

"So far as behaviors go, mother-infant cosleeping is one of the few primate universals. The main exceptions are found in a relatively small subset of human primates, among Western, Educated, Industrialized, Rich, and Democratic societies, sometimes referred to as WEIRD. In this comprehensive, humane, very clear, and also brave book, James McKenna strives to renormalize our segment of humanity."

>—Sarah Blaffer Hrdy, Ph.D., author of *Mother Nature* and *Mothers and Others: The Evolutionary Origins of Mutual Understanding*

"In this book, Professor McKenna distills his decades of anthropological work on normal human infant sleep into an accessible form. His clear explanations on the importance of nighttime closeness and 'breastsleeping' in human evolution and culture, paired with practical guidance, are sure to empower and support families."

>—Cecilia Tomori, Ph.D., Assistant Professor of Anthropology, Durham University, Durham Infancy & Sleep Centre (DISC)

# SAFE INFANT SLEEP

## Expert Answers to Your Cosleeping Questions

)

### JAMES J. MCKENNA, PH.D.

Forewords by
WILLIAM SEARS, M.D., and MEREDITH F. SMALL, PH.D.

With contributions from
PETER S. BLAIR, PH.D.

Platypus Media, LLC
Washington, D.C.

Safe Infant Sleep; Expert Answers to Your Cosleeping Questions
Written by James J. McKenna, Ph.D.
Illustrations by Alison Kreckmann
Additional Graphics by Hannah Thelen

Text © 2022, 2020: James J. McKenna
Illustrations and Additional Graphics © 2022, 2020: Platypus Media, LLC

Paperback ISBN-13: 978-1-930775-76-3
  First Edition • January 2020
  Second Edition • May 2022
eBook ISBN-13:  978-1-930775-77-0 • Available for Kindle, Sony, Kobo, and Nook

Audiobook produced by Tantor Media and available through major audiobook distributors

Available in Spanish as Sueño infantil seguro: Respuestas de los expertos a tus preguntas sobre el colecho
Paperback ISBN-13: 978-1-930775-68-8
eBook ISBN-13: 978-1-930775-53-4

Published in the United States by:
  Platypus Media, LLC
  750 First Street NE, Suite 700
  Washington, DC 20002
  202-546-1674 • Fax: 202-5558-2132
  www.PlatypusMedia.com • Info@PlatypusMedia.com

Distributed to the book trade in the United States by:
  National Book Network (North America)
    301-459-3366 • Toll-free: 800-462-6420
    CustomerCare@NBNbooks.com • NBNbooks.com
  NBN international (worldwide)
    NBNi.Cservs@IngramContent.com • Distribution.NBNi.co.uk

Library of Congress Cataloging-in-Publication Data
  McKenna, James J. (James Joseph), 1948-
  Safe infant sleep: expert answers to your cosleeping questions / James J. McKenna. — 1st ed.
    p. cm.
  Includes index.
  ISBN-13: 978-1-930775-76-3
  ISBN-10: 1-930775-76-8
  1. Co-sleeping. I. Title.
  Library of Congress Control Number: 2019950170

11 10 9 8 7 6 5 4 3 2

Printed in the United States of America

# Sleeping with Your Baby Around the World!

Dr. McKenna's research, insights, and data are reaching healthcare professionals and families across the globe. Platypus Media is proud that his previous cosleeping book has been translated into many languages!

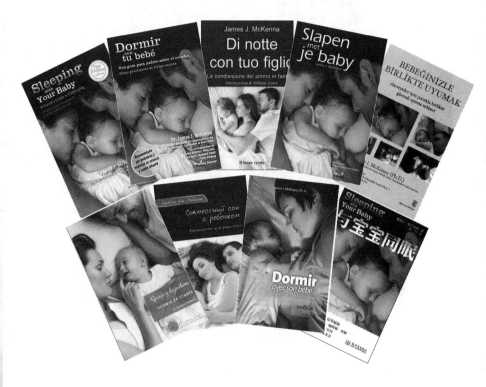

*Sleeping with Your Baby* (English)
*Dormir con tu bebé* (Spanish)
*Di notte con tuo figlio* (Italian)
*Slapen met je baby* (Dutch)
*Bebeğinizle Birlikte Uyumak* (Turkish)

*Spanje z dojenčkom* (Slovenian)
*Спим вместе с ребенком* (Russian)
*Dormir avec son bébé* (French)
与宝宝同眠 (Chinese)

- - - - - - - - - - - - - - - - - - - - - - - - -

All these editions are available on our website.
Visit us at www.PlatypusMedia.com

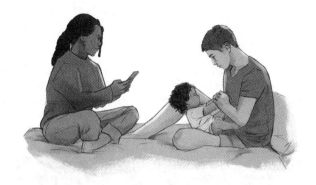

## EDITORIAL TEAM

Managing Editor:      Hannah Thelen, Silver Spring, MD

Senior Editor:        Dia L. Michels, Washington, D.C.

Associate Editors:    Alison Kreckmann, Washington, D.C.
                      Amy Nash, Denver, CO
                      Anna Cohen, Washington, D.C.
                      Anna Tippett, Fredericksburg, VA
                      Destany Atkinson, Washington, D.C.
                      Huneeya Siddiqui, Washington, D.C.
                      Jenelise Sutton, Washington, D.C.
                      Megan Shaffer, Bloomsburg, PA
                      Victoria Stingo, Washington, D.C.

## DESIGN TEAM

Cover Design:      Victoria Stingo, Washington, D.C.

Illustrations:     Alison Kreckmann, Washington, D.C.

Layout/Graphics:   Hannah Thelen, Silver Spring, MD

## SPECIAL THANKS TO

Peter J. Fleming, Ph.D., University of Bristol, U.K.
Helen L. Ball, Ph.D., Durham University, U.K.

# Dedication and Acknowledgements

Throughout my 30-year career studying human infants and mothers, and sleep and breastfeeding, I have had the remarkable privilege of engaging with, learning from, and witnessing inspirational generosity by midwives, doulas, lactation counselors, and lactation researchers—all women across the globe working quietly and selflessly on behalf of mothers, babies, and families. The commitment and kindnesses I have witnessed, alongside their skills and their intelligences, go well beyond what I can adequately describe. In a hierarchical system where appropriate recognition, financial rewards, and the level of respect they deserve is often missing, I dedicate this book to them and say thank you to each. It has been an honor to count you among my colleagues and friends, always reminding me to keep my eyes on those we are seeking to help.

I also dedicate this book to one of the most masterful, hardworking, organized, and creative partners I may have ever worked with, my editor, Hannah Thelen. I have never thought of my own writing as necessarily sub-par, but in a flash, Hannah could take something I wrote and turn it into magic, or certainly something more appealing and expressive than my own prose. Thank you, Hannah.

And to you, Dia, my publisher: while we haven't always seen eye-to-eye, you persisted anyway. I hope our partnership will have, at long last, produced an undeniable, scientifically-valued book that can successfully strike at the core of the traditional infant sleep paradigm. Together, perhaps we can begin to eliminate erroneous and hurtful ways of thinking that, for over a century, undermined (however unintended) the chances for infant survival and more optimal and enjoyable nighttime experiences for both infants and parents alike.

# Contents

# Part 6: Final Thoughts

# Appendices

> The great enemy of truth is very often not the lie—deliberate, contrived, and dishonest—but the myth—persistent, persuasive, and unrealistic. Too often we hold fast to the clichés of our forebears. We subject all facts to a prefabricated set of interpretations. We enjoy the comfort of opinion without the discomfort of thought.

—President John F. Kennedy, 1962
Yale University Commencement

# FOREWORD BY
# Meredith Small, Ph.D.

We live in fearful times, and nowhere is that fear more apparent than among parents, especially new parents. No matter that humans have been making little humans for at least 200,000 years, no matter that babies are born every second of every day and all around the world, every parent still worries about doing the "right thing" to guide their child toward competent adulthood. What brought on this collective parental anxiety?

Some of that fear comes from inexperience. The birth rate in Western culture has been decreasing over the last 50 years, and, as a result, many of us parents have no idea what we are doing. There are fewer brothers and sisters to practice on and fewer babysitting jobs. Many people, especially in the United States, also move away from their own parents and extended families, which means it often feels like one is bringing up children solo, even with a partner involved. As families have grown smaller, there are also fewer opportunities to learn from and correct mistakes with each successive kid. Instead, our eggs are in one basket, which makes us obsess about that basket. Who should we ask, then, when needing parenting advice?

> Parenting advice has been more destructive than helpful. Many mothers today express exasperation because one "expert" contradicts the next "expert."

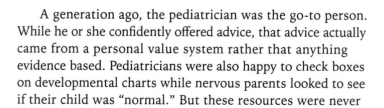

A generation ago, the pediatrician was the go-to person. While he or she confidently offered advice, that advice actually came from a personal value system rather that anything evidence based. Pediatricians were also happy to check boxes on developmental charts while nervous parents looked to see if their child was "normal." But these resources were never very good; training for pediatricians is medical not behavioral, and the charts are there to catch outliers, not the wide range of possibilities and the even wider time frame in which these developmental stages might appear.

Many anxious parents also turned to parenting advice books, and what a barrage of conflicting information that has been! Bookstores and libraries are filled with shelf after shelf of advice books telling parents what to do and judging them if they decide to go a different way. Others have been snowed under by the internet. Blogs abound on every single move a baby or parent makes, and these are written by people who only have experience with their own children, yet they are dogmatic that there is only one good way to parent.

This flurry of parenting advice has been more destructive than helpful. Many mothers today express exasperation because one "expert" contradicts the next "expert." Some mothers become anxious, depressed, and have feelings of inadequacy. I don't think it's a coincidence that this judgmental atmosphere around the arena that women naturally "owned" (that is, motherhood), came on the heels of the feminist revolution. I'd call it a punishing backlash. In that sense, any decision a woman might make as a new parent that flies in the face of the judgmental advice books, the hysterical and critical internet pundits, inflexible pediatricians, and strident governmental recommendations are, in fact, feminist issues.

The best antidote to all this? Choose your "experts" wisely.

And so, we turn to Dr. James McKenna, because he is a truly trustworthy expert. He has first-hand experience as a father, a scientist, a sleep physiology expert, an evolutionary biologist who knows the long history of our species, a social anthropologist familiar with cross-cultural examples, and a historian probing into the specific issue of parent-infant sleep over generations. In other words, Dr. McKenna is not relying on some opinion he conjured out of thin air, but real live data and research. His data are also supported, in the most scholarly and broad way, by evolutionary, historical, and cross-cultural theory. That's why Dr. McKenna has earned a kind of credibility that is rare, even unheard of, in the world of parenting advice.

But more than that, Dr. McKenna is not the kind of academic who is happy to sit safely in his ivory tower. Instead, he faces and considers, with data and deep thought, every challenge to cosleeping that the governmental authorities and the internet cough up. While we might admire his knowledge and experience, it is his persistence in promoting cosleeping, and now breastsleeping, that is his best gift to parents and to our culture. Dr. McKenna never stops learning, never stops thinking about all this, and sometimes it seems he is the only expert out there who still has the emotional and psychological health of parents and babies as his main focus. He doesn't ever tell parents what to do; he judges no one. Instead, as *Safe Infant Sleep* shows, he lays out all the evidence and then lets families decide what is best for them.

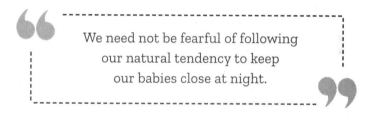

> We need not be fearful of following our natural tendency to keep our babies close at night.

Dr. McKenna's previous book, *Sleeping With Your Baby* (2007), focused on cosleeping and his work over the years as well as providing clear answers to question about where babies "should" sleep and why. The current book is not merely an updated version of that book. In *Safe Infant Sleep*, Dr. McKenna introduces the new—and yet somehow intuitive—idea that babies and moms sleep best, and more naturally, when they are together and there is easy access to the breast all night long. This current book is also full of answers to questions about SIDS and cosleeping, how fathers fare in the cosleeping system, and how belief systems, such as inherent racism, cloud what should be a simple decision to lie down and sleep with your child. And, in a conversational way, Dr. McKenna brings us all up to date on the most current research in this area.

In that sense, *Safe Infant Sleep* is not just a parenting guide, or maybe it's just an unusual one. It breaks apart every single issue about infant sleep that a mother or father might question as they start their life's journey with their baby. But take heed—the kind of thoroughness and thoughtfulness you see here should be the template you demand when asking other so-called experts about parenting issues.

Yes, we live in fearful times, but because of Dr. James McKenna, we need not be fearful of following our natural tendency to keep our babies close at night. Read this book and become informed, and then pick up your baby, crawl in bed with them (or don't), and sleep safely.

❱

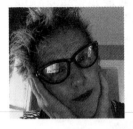

MEREDITH F. SMALL is a writer, Professor Emerita of Anthropology at Cornell University, and Visiting Scholar in the Department of Anthropology at the University of Pennsylvania.

She received a Ph.D. in Biological Anthropology from the University of California, Davis, and spent several years studying the behavior of macaque monkeys in captivity and in the wild.

Her work has appeared in *Discover, Natural History, Scientific American,* and *New Scientist,* among many other magazines and newspapers. Small was also a regular commentator for National Public Radio's *All Things Considered.* She is the author of five books, including *Kids* and *Our Babies, Ourselves.*

# FOREWORD BY
# William Sears, M.D.

You are about to read groundbreaking research from not only the leading scientist in the world of mother-baby sleep, but also a passionate father who has devoted most of his professional life to studying the practice of cosleeping.

One of the most memorable moments in my professional life as a pediatrician was my first meeting with Dr. McKenna in Pasadena, CA, in 1982. At that time, my wife Martha had been, shall we say, doing what comes naturally—cosleeping with our babies. We learned about nighttime parenting literally on the job. Our first three babies slept well in their own cribs, either in our bedroom or in their own room, but babies four and five needed a nighttime upgrade.

I still remember the night Martha woke up to the I-need-you-mommy cries of our one-month-old baby, Hayden, and Martha said, from her heart, "I don't care what the books say. I've got to get some sleep!" She instinctively put Hayden next to her in the bed to breastfeed, and the pair slept happily thereafter. While watching this beautiful nighttime parenting scenario, I was struck by the thought that this is the way it was meant to be.

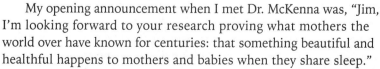

> The way mothers and babies get to know one another through shared sleep is too valuable to be left to opinion.

My opening announcement when I met Dr. McKenna was, "Jim, I'm looking forward to your research proving what mothers the world over have known for centuries: that something beautiful and healthful happens to mothers and babies when they share sleep."

When he began his research as a Professor of Anthropology and Director of the Mother-Baby Behavioral Sleep Laboratory at the University of Notre Dame, parenting books were full of misinformation from unreliable sources about cosleeping. But the way mothers and babies get to know one another through shared sleep is too valuable to be left to opinion. Many of today's savvy parents smartly ask, "Show me the science!" In *Safe Infant Sleep*, Dr. McKenna does just that.

His research takes you on a journey into the brains and bodies of mothers and babies when they share sleep, with my favorite novel feature of this book being Dr. McKenna's insightful use of the term "breastsleeping." Through his scientific experiments, Dr. McKenna shows that this style of nighttime parenting is the way mommy brains and baby brains are wired to experience sleep, and proves how and why bedsharing can be safe.

> Rather than scare new parents away
> from sleeping with their babies,
> healthcare providers should be teaching
> strategies for safe cosleeping.

As you will learn throughout these chapters, cosleeping is also co-smartening. Consider your baby's brain like a growing garden. Safe cosleeping is the perfect "gardener" during the window of opportunity that is the first two years—when a baby's brain is growing the fastest, building neurological pathways that give a child a healthy start into a life of mental wellness.

With insights from the most up-to-date research, you will read how safe cosleeping, in all its forms, reduces infant cerebral stress, programming these growing little brains to be able to better manage stress later in life.

While reading this guide to happy, healthy, and safe cosleeping, or—better said—breastsleeping, get ready to think, "Oh, this validates my intuition!" That's what a book that is science- and experience-based should do, unlike the many nighttime parenting guides that actually confuse moms about cosleeping. One piece of mommy-wisdom that I describe daily in my practice is to ask yourself, when deciding how to react to any parenting situation, if I were my baby, how would I want my mother to react? That natural, maternal instinct reaction would be to pick up your fussy baby, snuggle together, and breastsleep. Ahhh… that was simple!

Rather than scare new parents away from sleeping with their babies, healthcare providers should be teaching strategies for safe cosleeping. Dr. McKenna lists time-tested and scientifically-studied methods of sleeping safely with your baby. He provides hope for a future that embraces the positive potential of cosleeping, and helps parents feel empowered to choose the right sleeping arrangement for their family.

Imagine you're among a group of smart new parents I call "high investors." You seek consultation with the top doc in your area on the newest science about infant care. You open your consultation with, "Doctor, what is one simple parenting choice I can make that could have lasting mental and physical health benefits?" In the world that Dr. McKenna is fighting to create, she would get out her prescription pad and write: "Breastsleep with your baby."

*Safe Infant Sleep* is a must-read for every expectant and new parent, and belongs in the required reading library of every babycare advisor. If babies could talk, they would shout, "Thanks, Mom, for reading this book and for keeping me safe and sound!"

❭

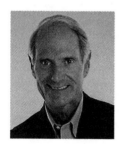

DR. WILLIAM SEARS, or Dr. Bill as his "little patients" call him, has been advising parents on how to raise healthier families for over 40 years. He received his medical training at Harvard Medical School's Children's Hospital in Boston and The Hospital for Sick Children in Toronto, before serving as the chief of pediatrics at Toronto Western Hospital. He has served as a professor of pediatrics at several universities.

Together with his wife Martha, he has written more than 40 best-selling books and countless articles on nutrition, parenting, and healthy aging. He serves as a health consultant for magazines, TV, radio and other media, and his AskDrSears.com website is one of the most popular health and parenting sites. Dr. Sears has appeared on over 100 television programs, including 20/20, Good Morning America, Oprah, Today, The View, and Dr. Phil, and was featured on the cover of *TIME Magazine* in May 2012.

# Read This First:
## A Note from the Author

The question of whether or not to sleep with your baby is complicated. It does not lend itself to easy answers or catchy slogans. As new parents, you are typically faced with cosleeping conundrums in the middle of the night when exhaustion is high, and what works for your family may conflict with what you have been taught about sleep safety by your pediatrician. In addition, there are racial, class, social, and political biases that run through cosleeping data, and the advice you get from many healthcare providers is often based on accepted practice instead of accurate, evidence-based research.

It is a shame that new parents need to read an entire book just to be able to sleep soundly at night, but this seems to be the case. When it comes to sleep, knowing what you are doing and why you are doing it can help everyone feel well-rested, provide physical and emotional benefits for babies, and even save lives.

> I ask that you take the time to read this entire book to fully understand the topic, as well as your options, so you can make safe, informed choices.

Parents ask me for advice all the time, and it is hard to give it because each home is different, each set of parents has different goals, and each child has different needs. I want each family to make the decision that is appropriate for them. I ask that you take the time to read this entire book to fully understand the topic, as well as your options, so you can make safe, informed choices.

While I have tried to provide comprehensive information and varied perspectives, you may notice as you read that there are many questions remaining that have yet to be researched. Humans can be complicated. When it comes to family sleep, there are a plethora of sleeping arrangements and outside factors that can affect sleep safety. It is frustrating to me that some of the questions parents ask simply do not have answers yet.

It is up to influential health organizations to decide which questions are worth investigating and, by extension, which research projects deserve funding in order to find answers. When the subject is controversial, like bedsharing or other infant sleep issues, these decisions are subject to systemic bias. Unfortunately, research priorities are based on a flawed infant sleep paradigm that is inherently in conflict with cosleeping, so these organizations tend to ignore the many questions we still have about how to cosleep safely. Most studies simply aim to find evidence that validates the views of those making the decisions.

Part of the goal of this book, which encourages nonjudgmental discussions about cosleeping, is to open the door for future studies by encouraging health professionals to make the process of deciding research priorities more inclusive. It is my hope that public health authorities will one day be able to address the many questions we still have, and, in doing so, be able to provide the best possible recommendations tailored to individual families.

The biggest question on your mind at the moment is likely, "Where should my baby sleep?" I hope you will not be disappointed to find that I can't answer that question for you, and neither can any pediatrician, healthcare institution, or researcher. This decision is only yours to make, and should be based on a thorough understanding of the risks and benefits, your overall family circumstances, and the parameters of your sleep space. External medical authorities don't know you, your infant, or the needs, wants, and values of your family.

My sincere hope is that the information provided here will place you in the best possible position to decide the answer of where your baby should sleep for yourself. If this book leads you to understand that you and your family will come to know your baby better than anyone, and that your baby will ultimately teach you what he or she needs to make him or her (and you) healthier and happier, I will view it as a success.

# Breastsleeping:
## What It Means and Why It's Important

*"This concept is a potential game-changer given the current polarized debate on what we should be advising parents...."*

—DR. KATHLEEN A. MARINELLI, ET AL.[1]

*Breastsleeping* is a term recently coined by myself and my colleague, Dr. Lee T. Gettler. It refers to a specific kind of bedsharing between a breastfeeding mother and infant, occurring in an environment free from proven risk factors. It is the safest form of bedsharing, practiced worldwide for all of human history.

Breastsleeping is part of an evolved, diverse, and highly integrated set of human behaviors. It remains fundamental to the continuing health of our species, in addition to potentially optimizing the health of individual mothers and their infants in both the short and long term.

This sleeping arrangement not only provides more opportunities to breastfeed throughout each night, but also makes it more likely that mothers will breastfeed their infants for a greater number of months.

Breastsleeping enhances sensitivity between mother and infant, encourages lighter sleep (see Chapter 6), and reduces the risk of danger in a variety of other ways.[2, 3] Our primary aim in creating a new term for this very old concept is to provide a new research category that acknowledges three things:

1. The role that consistent maternal contact plays in helping to establish optimal breastfeeding.

2. The significant extent to which breastfeeding and nightly sensory exchanges change all aspects of mother-infant sleep compared to traditional solitary or bottle-fed infant sleep models.

3. That the unique behaviors and physiological characteristics exhibited by breastsleeping mothers and infants mean that breastsleeping must be given its own category for assessing potential benefits and risks.

After decades of studying bedsharing and infant health, it is clear that it is not possible to document biologically normal human infant sleep outside of the breastsleeping context. The ongoing sensory exchanges (of touch, sound, smell, and taste) between mother and infant during breastfeeding—and the breastmilk itself—significantly change infant and maternal sleep architecture, infant metabolism, the efficiency of the infant's immune system, and the infant's microbiome (helpful bacteria). Recent research also suggests positive changes to an infant's growing and expanding neural connections and overall brain architecture.[4, 5] These will all be discussed later in the book.

In the more immediate sense, breastsleeping is associated with an increase in brief waking periods and in breastmilk consumption, effects that enhance protection against sleep-related deaths and are altogether good for babies while being less disruptive for mothers.

# Part 1

## Cosleeping is Normal

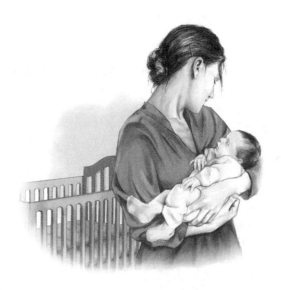

## CHAPTER 1

# Why I Care So Much About This Subject

*"There is no such thing as a baby, there is a baby and someone."*

—DONALD W. WINNICOTT[6]

Many of my friends find it amusing that I spend almost all my waking hours studying what people do when they sleep. It's true. What people do when they're asleep fascinates me—and not just people in general, but families in particular. At the University of California, Irvine Medical Center, and as Director of the Mother-Baby Behavioral Sleep Laboratory at the University of Notre Dame, my students and I have had the privilege of documenting information about infant sleep through infrared video recordings and physiological monitoring of mothers and infants sleeping both together and apart.

Our research was not just for the sake of gathering knowledge, but for helping mothers and infants sleep better, thrive physically and emotionally, and stay as safe as possible no matter where or how they choose to sleep.

When it comes to parenting, new moms and dads are flooded with conflicting advice from family members, well-meaning friends, medical professionals, the media, the government, and, of course, from other parents. The vast majority of parents want to do what is best for their children, yet this bombardment of information implies that parental wisdom and the capacity of parents to make their own informed decisions is somehow out of their grasp. It's as if everyone knows exactly what is best for your baby except for you!

It is not my intention to tell you what to do or how your infant should sleep. British author Christina Hardyment wrote: "Telling mothers and fathers how to bring up their children in books is arguably as silly as sending false teeth through the post and hoping they fit."[7] I would never wish to give you ill-fitting teeth, and I certainly don't wish to give you ill-fitting rules for how to be a good parent, as all families and their circumstances are different. What is good for one family may not be good for another. The purpose of this book is to provide the best information available in order to help you make your own choice about what sleeping arrangement will be the safest and most beneficial for your family.

My wife Joanne and I entered the world of parenting with the birth of our son, Jeffrey, in 1978. Anxious about our new set of responsibilities, we read book after book on parenting. We are both anthropologists and we were quite taken aback at what we found in the childcare literature. When it came to what the experts had to say about feeding patterns and sleeping arrangements, either all of our research and training about the universal aspects of human life was wrong, or the pediatric experts were missing or ignoring key information concerning what infants need most: specialized nutrition from breastmilk, and sustained physical contact both day and night.

Not only was there nothing in the childcare books that reflected what we know about our primate heritage and sleeping arrangements, there was also nothing that reflected current research on human infant biology and the role that maternal touch plays in promoting infant growth and well-being. We learned that infant care recommendations were not based on empirical laboratory or field studies of infants at all, nor on cross-cultural insights as to how human babies actually live around the world.[8]

Rather, they were based on 70- or 80-year-old cultural ideas, uniquely Western and historically novel. Recommendations followed the social values of mostly male physicians who not only had never changed a diaper, but had never—in any substantial way—associated with, or taken care of, their own infants.

These "parenting experts" preferred to define babies in terms of who they wanted the infants to become, and decided what was good for infants based on recent and sometimes arbitrary social values, such as autonomy and independence. They should have been thinking in terms of who infants actually are— little creatures who are very much dependent physiologically, socially, and psychologically on the presence of a caregiver to an unprecedented degree and for an unprecedented length of time compared to other mammals.

The more we delved into the history and research of infant sleep recommendations, the more we discovered that the prevailing childcare wisdom had little basis in science whatsoever.[9] This discovery changed my career.

When you look at the prevalence of cosleeping in the mammal world, and among different cultures and in different eras of human history, it is clear that cosleeping is universal through time and is practiced far and wide in many different ways.

For hundreds of thousands of years, up to and through our early historic periods, breastfeeding mothers have practiced what Dr. Lee Gettler and I call *breastsleeping*. Breastsleeping is our new term and concept for the highly integrated system of healthy infant sleep combined with healthy breastfeeding behavior.[2, 10]

The practice of breastsleeping consists of sleeping next to one's primarily breastfed baby, and lying the infant on his or her back for sleep (which facilitates breastfeeding). This is such a universal and widespread practice that most parents worldwide couldn't imagine asking where the baby should sleep, whether it is okay to sleep with the baby, what position the baby should sleep in, and how the baby should be fed.

My anthropological training, as well as my own intuition, told me that something this common had to be beneficial, but it has only been through extensive and rigorous scientific study that we have determined why this proves to be the case.

During the '90s at the University of California Irvine School of Medicine Sleep Disorders Laboratory, my colleagues Drs. Sarah Mosko, Chris Richards, Claiborne Dungy, Sean Drummond, and

I conducted the first research on the physiology and behavior of breastsleeping mothers and babies.[11]

In one intensive three-year study, we examined infant and maternal sleep architecture, nighttime breastfeeding and its relationship with bedsharing, and the differences between infants who cosleep in the form of bedsharing and infants who sleep alone in separate rooms.

Our two preliminary studies, and subsequent related studies, employed rigorous scientific methods and analysis; our grant proposal earned a near-perfect score from one the most exclusive scientific grants in the U.S., offered by the National Institute of Child Health and Human Development (NICHD). We were also awarded the prestigious Shannon Award from the NICHD for our proposal's innovations and scientific promise. The research papers were then accepted by some of the most well-respected medical journals in the world.

Nighttime behavioral studies have continued at the University of Notre Dame Mother-Baby Behavioral Sleep Laboratory, where we have clearly demonstrated the special abilities of both low- and high-risk mothers to respond to their infants' needs while breastsleeping. Over time, other scientists began to study these same issues, affirming the validity of our research while adding many new insights.[12, 13, 14, 15, 16, 17]

Watching the peaceful sleep of an infant, it may appear that not much happens while they are snoozing; the infant's body simply requires downtime several times each day. And, yes, downtime functions to help one regain energy, but much more is going on. During sleep, all manner of physical and neurological processes, including developing inter-connections between new cells, are taking place. While infants sleep, the brain is sorting out how many and which brain cells will be retained, and where in the brain they need to go. This affects memory formation as well as intellectual, emotional, and psychological aspects of development.

During the first three to four months of life, the prefrontal cortex is invaded with young neurons taking shape and finding their place based on what the infant experiences on a daily basis.[18] The young brains of human infants need to "prune," or reduce, the nutrient demand of cells that don't seem to be used very often, so that vital nutrients can be shifted to more active cells. Your baby's engagements with you, even in this early time, are as developmentally important as going to school. They are learning and shaping their brains every step of the way, even while they sleep.

Without stimulation from contact and social interactions— including nighttime sensory exchanges—neonatal brain cells are potentially lost forever. This has led some developmental psychologists to argue that infants are far more threatened by what they do not receive in terms of neurological excitation than by what they do receive, since "pruned" infant brain cells are not retrievable at a later date. Minimizing contact with the mother's body can make an infant's neurological scaffolding less stable and effective, weakening the structures that provide the basis for the infant's rapidly growing communication skills, emotionality, and ability to effectively regulate and respond to his or her own needs.[19]

It is unfortunate that, in light of all of this new information, parents who sleep with their infants are often considered needy or deficient, or sometimes even irresponsible, by medical authorities. When we hear about babies who do not or cannot sleep alone through the night, rarely do we hear: *What a good baby!* even though that is exactly what is in a human infant's biological best interest.

The good news is that, as of 2016, the American Academy of Pediatrics (AAP) recommends that infants never sleep in separate rooms from their caregivers. The bad news is that they argue against sleeping in the same bed. Herein lies the controversy.

I wrote my first book on cosleeping in 2007, and now I want to offer an updated version with a bit more science in it. I want to share with you what I (and others) have learned about various forms of cosleeping and breastfeeding in the years since then, and why a combination of the two refuses to go away in spite of anti-bedsharing recommendations. I want families to understand how much happens during cosleeping, including critical communication between infants and mothers (and other caregivers) through touch, scent, sound, and taste. This unconscious sensory communication is part of the way our species has evolved to maximize health and survival. It is likewise an intrinsic part of the way parents communicate and experience love for and with their infants and each other. A baby sleeping on his or her own, outside the supervision of a caregiver, is deprived of this vital communication and, as scientific studies prove, is at risk on many different levels.

Cosleeping is not only normal, common, and instinctive, but it can also be in the best interest of a family when it is adopted for purposes of protecting and nurturing infants, when safety is given priority, and when the right kind of cosleeping is chosen for and by each unique family.

That being said, one cannot be naïve regarding the different ways in which people live. Families make different decisions and things don't always go according to plan. Good intentions can be waylaid by fatigue and shifting circumstances. While the ideal cosleeping environment is an exclusively breastfeeding mother sleeping on a flat surface that has been maximized for safety (we'll dig into this later), this ideal is not always the reality. There is no guarantee that anything we do with infants will necessarily be done in a safe way. Cosleeping in the form of bedsharing is no different. It is quite true that bedsharing can be practiced in ways that are dangerous. Bedsharing is generally a more complex and less stable practice than crib sleeping, which itself has both advantages and disadvantages for babies.

> One size does not fit all when it comes to sleeping arrangements.

I want to teach families to avoid known risks in any sleeping arrangement. Being aware of where dangers lie and what can and cannot be modified is critical. One size does not fit all when it comes to sleeping arrangements, and where households exhibit risk factors for dangerous bedsharing, I encourage alternative sleep practices.

No sleep environment is completely risk free, but the fact that a bedsharing environment cannot be made 100% risk free is no more an argument for a global recommendation against all bedsharing than it is an argument for a global recommendation against all crib sleeping—because crib sleeping incurs risks too, evidenced by the continuing epidemic of Sudden Infant Death Syndrome (SIDS).

To use a different example, consider that thousands of people die from choking while eating every year, even though eating is normal, common, and instinctive. In order to minimize the risks, adults are not advised to stop eating (which would be silly) but instead are instructed to learn the Heimlich maneuver, as well as specialized food preparation and feeding techniques for young children. Similarly, we learn with great effort how to properly use and place infants in car seats, yet many babies die each year in cars due to some parents' disregard for ways to minimize car travel risks. Still, it would be impractical and unreasonable to ban automobile transportation for children altogether.

This book is intended to provide a balanced, comprehensive, and holistic perspective on cosleeping and bedsharing. It is intended to provide safety information and reassurance to those families who are considering or who currently choose to sleep with their babies. Enjoying every minute with your baby—whether you are awake or asleep—is important. Though it might not seem like it at first, our time with them is very short.

I hope that this book will enable you to feel comfortable holding, carrying, and responding to your baby, and will help you feel good about your caregiving choices. I know I am not alone in wanting to help you and your family thrive and enjoy experiences that can be cherished forever.

My intention is not to convince everyone to bedshare. The point is simply that the real answer to the question of whether or not any particular family should bedshare is always: *It depends.* While it is safe and appropriate to recommend that no infant should sleep alone in a separate room from an adult caregiver, this is just the starting point. Beyond that, there are many factors to consider before choosing a sleeping arrangement. I hope this book will give you the specific knowledge you need to make an informed decision, as well as the confidence to assess your conditions and circumstances in order to choose both what feels right and is safe for you and your family.

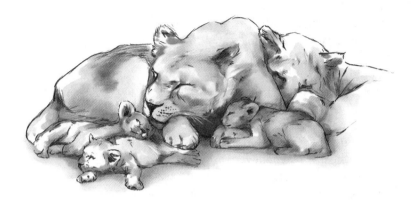

CHAPTER 2

# What Is Cosleeping?

## Cosleeping vs. Breastsleeping

Many people don't fully understand the term "cosleeping," but they use it nonetheless because they have a sense of what it means. Picture a mother lion and her cubs sleeping in a big heap, paws on top of backs, heads on bellies, body parts rising and falling with each rhythmic breath, the whole group intertwined in one peaceful lump of warmth and touching. That is cosleeping, or at least one version of it.

Cosleeping refers to the many different ways babies or children sleep in close emotional and physical contact with their families, usually within arm's reach. Whether it is for protection, warmth, ease of nursing, or comfort, humans and other mammals routinely sleep side-by-side, generation after generation. In one way or another, cosleeping remains universal for our species, predating history itself.

This book is both about cosleeping, as practiced in Western cultures and around the globe, and a specific form of cosleeping that I have come to refer to as breastsleeping.

General cosleeping cannot necessarily be characterized the same way across all situations. For example, as former Florida State University football coach Bobby Bowden once said in the South Bend Tribune, "I slept in the same bed with my granddaddy...then in the same bed with my four cousins. I never slept alone until I got married." And my friend and colleague Dr. Robert Hahn at the Centers for Disease Control and Prevention (CDC) once defined cosleeping for me in this way: "Cosleeping is when my two lovely daughters are sleeping at the same time."[20]

While each family's circumstances may vary, they can all be said to "cosleep" whenever they cuddle, snuggle, and snooze together close enough to detect and respond to each other—whether on the same surface or not. Of course, this doesn't tell you about what forms of cosleeping are safe or unsafe, which will be made clear later.

Breastsleeping, however, is clearly defined. Perhaps the safest form of cosleeping, breastsleeping is specifically comprised of a breastfeeding mother-baby pair sharing a bed during sleep in order to facilitate breastfeeding. As you will discover throughout this book, breastsleeping is one of the most beneficial forms of cosleeping for mother and baby. If practiced safely (see Chapter 8), breastsleeping may protect against SIDS, help the whole family get a little more sleep, and make important contributions to an infant's development in the first year of life.

> It is not possible to document biologically normal human infant sleep outside of the breastsleeping context.

It is very important to acknowledge that the term "cosleeping" does not exclusively refer to bedsharing and breastsleeping, but also encompasses roomsharing, or any situation in which parents and infants are within arms' reach but not necessarily sleeping on the same surface. Given the variety of behaviors that fall under the cosleeping umbrella, we are faced with the difficult task of agreeing that, while not all forms of cosleeping are safe, not all forms of cosleeping are dangerous either. For example, some medical authorities mistakenly state that cosleeping is dangerous, when they really mean to say that couch or sofa cosleeping is dangerous (which is always true), or that bedsharing is dangerous (which may or may not be true, depending on how it is practiced).

To speak about cosleeping without specifying the type of cosleeping is to create more controversy and confusion than necessary. While there may still be differences of opinion as to how to read the scientific findings on bedsharing, there is generally much more agreement on some of these issues than there might appear to be based on conflicting uses of the terminology.

There is no one right way to cosleep, nor does cosleeping occur in one correct configuration. One thing is for sure— regardless of whether or not you sleep on the same or a different surface, or in the same or a different room, remember that no one knows your baby better than you, and no one can anticipate and respond to the immediate needs of your baby as well as you. I like to point out that forms of cosleeping are likely as diverse as the cultures practicing them.

Regardless of where you're from, or your income, educational background, or social status, keeping a baby close and nursing throughout the night are simple ways of meeting a child's needs. Families have shared sleep on flat futons, mats, mattresses, and in hammocks. Some cosleepers lie next to each other on the floor. Some Americans who breastsleep lay a mattress in the center of the room away from walls; if a parent chooses to bedshare, this is likely the safest way to do it. Others sleep in the same room with the adult on a bed and the baby in a bassinet or crib a few feet away. Still others fall asleep in individual rooms, and then come together in the middle of the night (when it is time for a feeding or the baby has awoken and wants to be near an adult).

Cosleeping can be an ever-evolving process—babies may move from a crib, where they are placed at the beginning of the night, to their parent's bed, to a bassinet, and back again. Your baby may fall asleep in your bed and stay there all night, fall asleep in your bed and be moved later during sleep, or fall asleep elsewhere and be welcomed in for a feeding in the middle of the night—or you may fall asleep in the baby's room and sleep some or all of the night there.

Cosleeping can be practiced the same way, night after night, or can vary and shift as the baby grows and the family's needs change. My discussions with thousands of parents through the years tell me that there is not just one environment within which an infant sleeps, but several. All of this variability illustrates what parents of newborns quickly discover—their baby's sleep patterns are subject to frequent change, and sometimes it is hard to predict where exactly any given baby will sleep. As babies experience teething, they may have a difficult time sleeping. As newborns grow into older babies and toddlers, their cognitive and emotional development will affect their nighttime needs (see Chapter 10). As infants begin to place meaning on their daily experiences (some of them frightening), they might need more comforting to help them deal with increased confusion and nightmares. During times of stress, being close throughout the night is especially reassuring for your child.

Sharing sleep with babies is natural for most families in non-industrialized cultures, but families in industrialized societies must often "relearn" specific methods of cosleeping. In other words, most of us have very little experience with cosleeping, as our own parents likely did not practice it, leaving us unprepared.

It is true that we need to be very conscious of how we cosleep. If bedsharing, bedding and furniture arrangements and the sleeping arrangements of other children or pets must be taken into consideration. In order to protect and promote the well-being of your baby, you will need to be aware of safe cosleeping strategies, particularly if you choose to breastsleep. How and where your family chooses to cosleep can be adapted, though, or modified, to what you and your baby need in order to sleep as comfortably and as safely as possible.

Creating a safe cosleeping environment for your infant may require considerable effort, but these efforts can lead to enormous rewards. It is important to consider the positive impact that the type of cosleeping you choose can have on establishing and maintaining a close bond (especially for parents who are away from their baby many hours during the day), and how it is especially beneficial in supporting the breastfeeding relationship.

Now, and throughout history, cosleeping has played an important role in promoting infant survival and well-being, and has always made both short- and long-term contributions to healthy development.

# How the Animals Do It— What Happens When Deprived of It

*"For species such as primates, the mother is the environment."*

—DR. SARAH BLAFFER HRDY[21]

Mammals instinctually remain close to their young. Their babies would not survive for very long without the warmth, food, protection, and psychological nourishment their mothers provide. While mammals in general develop through their life stages at remarkably different rates, all mammals cosleep in one form or another. When and how this takes place, however, varies according to how each species has adapted to their environment and what kind of niche they fill in their habitat, including what they do there and how they eat, avoid predation, adapt to the climate, mate, give birth, and care for their young. Also of critical importance are the mother's ecological adaptations, including her relationship to the males and other group members, and her own nutritional, maintenance, and energy requirements.

For example, primates (including humans) typically give birth to one offspring at a time, providing each infant the opportunity to sleep alone with the mother or father. Primates depend on learning skills in a social context, so single births allow each infant to receive maximum attention during their very long and vulnerable infancy. Human infants in particular are in need of a great deal of contact, emotional support, breastfeeding, and transportation, for a very long time.

Some animal mothers (such as polar bears and migrating whales) fast while the babies are young, using their stores of body fat to sustain themselves and produce breastmilk for their young. Others (like lions) share the tasks of childminding and hunting so that the community ensures that both tasks get done. A significant number of mammal mothers leave their young hidden away (beneath low-lying shrubs, up in trees, or in dens, burrows, caves, or lairs) while they forage for the food they need to sustain themselves and to make milk for their babies. These mammals are called the "nested species."

The babies of these nested species do not cry when their mothers leave, in part because predators would be able to hear and track them, but mostly because their mothers' milk is so rich in fat that, after nursing, they remain satisfied during their mothers' absence. For example, fawns are hidden in nests beneath bushes and remain alone for periods as long as eight to ten hours. Deer milk is 19% fat, allowing these babies to stay full until their mother returns. Then, the babies will nurse again and the entire family, including the mother and siblings, will sleep nestled together.

Unlike these nested species, primate mammals, such as monkeys, apes, and humans, are referred to by scientists as the "carrying species." Our milk contains more water and sugar, less protein, and about 10%–20% less fat than that of the nested species. Fat is the growth nutrient, and mammals with low fat content in their breastmilk grow at a slower rate than those mammals who drink fat-rich milk. Fat is also what keeps you full, so after nursing, primate mammals are only satisfied for

## How Biology of Mother's Milk Predicts Mothering Behavior

| Nested Species (Feed and Leave) | Carrying Species (Cosleeping) |
| --- | --- |
| Ungulates (hoofed mammals) | Humans and other primates |
| High in fat<br>High in protein<br>Low in carbohydrates | Low in fat<br>Low in protein<br>High in carbohydrates |
| High calories = long interval between feeds | Low calories = short interval between feeds |
| To avoid predators, nested infants do not defecate or cry in the mother's absence | Carried infants cry in the absence of the mother and defecate spontaneously |

*Fig. 1.1 Some species are designed to be left by their mothers in their nest or burrow for many hours at a time. Others, like humans, need to be carried and in continuous contact with their mothers. Feeding freqency correlates with the composition of breastmilk, particularly the density of calories delivered by the mother per breastfeed.*

one or two hours before they need to eat again to eliminate their hunger. This need to breastfeed frequently means that primate mammals, in contrast to babies of the nesting species, must stay close to their mothers. Hence, rather than being safely tucked away somewhere, primate infants are carried until they reach at least 6–12 months of age, and usually until they are much older.

## Percentage of Adult Brain Size

| Age | Chimpanzee Infant | Human Infant |
|---|---|---|
| At birth | 45% | 25% |
| 3 months | 50% | 35% |
| 6 months | 60% | 45% |
| 9 months | 65% | 50% |
| 1 year | 70% | 60% |
| 2 years | 75% | 70% |
| 4 years | 85% | 80% |
| 8–9 years | 100% | 95% |

Fig. 1.2 Humans are born with only 25% of their adult brain size, which is less than any other mammal, and human infants take an exceptionally long time to reach adulthood.

Primate babies will sleep in their mothers' arms or while clinging to their backs, so that the infant becomes integrated into almost every aspect of the mother's daily routine.

This constant physical contact ensures that a physiological as well as a social bond is established between mother and baby, one that enables the neurologically immature primate newborn to develop and function more efficiently.

For us carrying species, then, the parents have an especially significant role in making growth possible. When an infant monkey is separated from its mother, the baby suffers—it experiences lower body temperature, an irregular heart rhythm, higher stress levels, and will, in extreme cases, become so clinically depressed that it eventually dies.

Human infants are born more helpless than any other primate, or any other animal species in the world. Most mammals are born with 60–90% of adult brain size. Humans, in contrast, are born with just 25% of their adult brain size. Our puny brain volume at birth explains why we are unable to cling to our mother's chests for easy transportation the way monkey and ape babies do. Compared with other mammals, human infants take the longest time to grow up, and they remain in a biologically dependent state for the longest period of time. Basically, compared to all other mammalian species, we are born premature.[22]

As the least neurologically mature primates, fed with breastmilk that is especially low in fat, human infants depend on care from an adult. Humans have even evolved traits that encourage adults to respond to an infant's needs, including some of our most unique, endearing attributes, like unparalleled empathy and generosity. Contributing to what some call the "help instinct," these traits likely developed for the sake of keeping our exceptionally vulnerable infants and children alive through exceptionally long periods of dependence.[23]

There is no such thing as giving a human infant too much contact or affection—humans thrive on touch, and the more an infant gets of it, the more they grow![24] When deprived of these sensations, a baby will use his or her primary survival response—crying—and will produce cortisol, a stress hormone, in an attempt to attract the attention of the parents.

Physical contact compensates for the fact that newborn humans cannot shiver to keep themselves warm and are unable to produce sufficient antibodies (that are present in mothers' milk) to protect them from illness. The sensation of touch itself stimulates the release of endorphins that help a baby's immature gut absorb the calories needed for growth. Developmental psychologist Dr. Tiffany Field found that human babies who were massaged 15 minutes per day experienced a remarkable 47% increase in daily weight gain compared with those infants who were not massaged.[25] Lots of contact is more than a nice social idea; it is what a healthy infant requires.

Human babies have been likened by anthropologist Dr. Ashley Montagu to little kangaroo joeys, which develop while fully insulated in their mothers' pouches. He says human infants are "extero-gestators,"[22] meaning they complete their gestation after birth, and someone's got to be there to help with it.

Dr. Montagu stresses that, like the kangaroo joey, the human infant's central nervous system depends on having a micro-environment that is similar to the maternal uterine environment from which it came, an environment full of sensory exchanges involving heat, sound, movement, transportation, feelings, touch, smells, and, of course, access to nutrients from the mother's breast.

As infants, human beings are not biologically designed nor prepared to be separated from their mothers. Separation can be tantamount to a death sentence.

---

*"The acceptance that we are primates and have many characteristics in common with other primates is no longer a particularly controversial concept....What is perhaps so surprising is that, until relatively recently, this concept was almost completely absent from most professional advice about infant care. This book goes a long way to correct this historical imbalance, and to help explain how our evolution as a species needs to be considered in understanding the needs of, and environmental effects on, the care given to young infants.*
*Accepting that close and almost continuous contact between infant and primary caregiver is the historical and evolutionary norm for our species is a very important starting point for families trying to juggle the needs of their young infant whilst meeting the other demands in their 21st century lives."*

—DR. PETER J. FLEMING

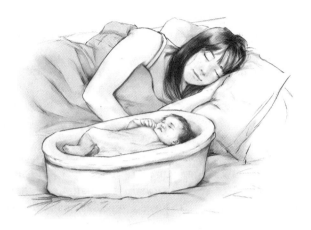

CHAPTER 3

# The History of Cosleeping

## Cosleeping Around the World

For the overwhelming majority of mothers and babies around the globe today, cosleeping is an unquestioned practice. In much of Southern Europe, Asia, Africa, Central America, and South America, mothers and babies routinely share sleep. In many cultures, cosleeping is the norm until children are weaned, and some continue long after weaning. Japanese parents (or grandparents) often sleep in proximity with their children until they are teenagers. They refer to this arrangement as a river, based on the character with the same meaning: 川. The mother is one bank, the father another, and the child sleeping between them is the water. Most of the present world cultures practice forms of cosleeping and there are very few cultures in the world that would have ever thought it acceptable or desirable to have babies sleeping alone.

For all of the cultures that cosleep regularly, there are an equal number of ways to practice it. Each culture selects and takes advantage of materials or structures in the local environment from which the sleeping arrangements emerge.

Aboriginal infants from Australia cosleep with their parents on the same surface, without any furniture and with minimal bedding (on blankets or mats), nestled up to their mothers' bodies—as do the Gusii of Kenya and the Bhil of the Western Ghats, in India.[8] Flores infants of Indonesia and Gund infants of northern China cosleep next to their caregivers on bamboo benches, mats, or futons placed on an earthen floor, while the Semang of Malaysia cosleep on split bamboo mattresses slightly raised off the ground. The Nahaue of northwest India and the Cuna of Panama sleep with their babies in hammocks strung up between two trees. Babies are placed in baskets hanging from the ceiling and lowered to arm's reach of their mothers by the Ainu of Japan from North Hokkaido and the Yapese island people.

In Pacific Micronesia, still other infants cosleep in the form of roomsharing. This also occurs in many Western cultures when infants remain within sensory access of their parents but sleep on different surfaces, like a bassinet, cradle, or crib.[26, 27] Another option, and a great compromise between roomsharing and bedsharing, is using a cosleeping device. These are crib-like extensions that can attach to the parents' bed, and are open on one side to allow you to slip the infant in and out for easy breastfeeding.[28]

Most cultures that routinely practice cosleeping, in any form, have very low rates of Sudden Infant Death Syndrome (SIDS). SIDS occurrences are among the lowest world-wide in Hong Kong, where cosleeping is extremely common.

Cosleeping is also more common in the U.S. than most people believe. The typical American home has a nursery for the baby, and parents report that the baby sleeps in a crib. Yet when researchers ask specific questions about who sleeps where, it turns out that the majority of mothers sleep with their young children at least part of most nights. Parents present themselves as having babies who sleep alone, following the societal norm of the baby in the baby's room and the couple in their own bedroom, but that is not an accurate representation of what is really happening in American homes.

Cosleeping is not unusual for American families at all. Studies report widely varying numbers of mothers who bedshare regularly, but it is typically between 25 and 80 percent. Regardless of the actual number, it is still clear that a large portion of mothers in the U.S. feel the powerful biological call to sleep in proximity to their infants. It would seem that the practice of bedsharing does not necessarily vary a great deal from culture to culture, but rather the social acceptance of it varies.

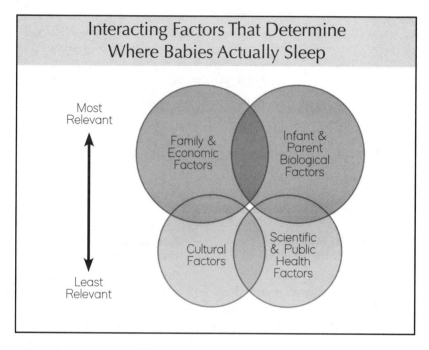

*Fig. 1.3 There are four main factors that determine where an infant sleeps, and these factors differ in significance among countries, cultures, and individual families.*

## Cultural and Historical Factors
## Leading to Modern Beliefs About Infant Sleep

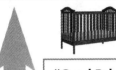

# Solitary Infant Sleep

### "Good Baby" Syndrome
Connected to previous factors, the distorted belief that an infant's moral character is tied to their sleep behavior deemed a baby to be "good" if they sleep through the night on their own.

### Technology is King
The belief in the superiority of new technology led parents to discount the nurturing power of human interaction and contact.

### Scientific Parenting
The rise of medical authoritative knowledge and caregiving "experts" reduced parental confidence in responding to their own instincts or knowledge of what their infant needs.

### Formula and Bottle-Feeding
The adoption of bottle-feeding and breastmilk substitutes made possible longer periods of sleep and separation for infants.

### Romanticized Relationships
The importance of romantic adult love emerged at the expense of prioritizing relationships with infants and children.

### The Rise of Individualism
Western values began to favor separation, autonomy, and self-sufficiency.

### Born Sinners
The concept of original sin made people believe infants were in need of cleansing and discipline.

### Intentional Overlaying
The Catholic church condemned bedsharing due to destitute women confessing to overlaying their babies on purpose.

*Fig. 1.4 The practice of infants sleeping alone in a crib was built upon layers of Western history, ideology, culture, and social norms.*

❯

# History of Infant Sleep in Western Industrialized Societies

Sleeping next to your child should instinctively be the most natural way for parents and babies to sleep. It is only in recent history that mothers, in the relatively small Western industrialized world, have had the dubious luxury to ask two basic questions: "How will my baby be fed?" and "Where will my baby sleep?"

No human ancestral or modern infant was ever separated from its caregiver, nocturnally or at any other time. What an odd notion for a mother to leave her helpless child all alone to sleep in an entirely separate space! Yet, today, people have been taught to be afraid of bedsharing. They have been warned that bedsharing will lead to parents unwittingly crushing their helpless infants, making moms and dads increasingly paranoid. How did we arrive at this unnatural conclusion?

There are a lot of reasons. Western fear of bedsharing can be traced all the way back to 500 years ago, in major European cities such as Paris, Brussels, Munich, and London. Historians have documented that Catholic priests in these cities condemned infants and parents sleeping in the same bed after poor women confessed to intentionally crushing their babies in bed in attempts to control family size.[29, 30] While this is an interesting historical factor to consider, there are also many pertinent cultural factors that more directly relate to our current condition.

First, there was the development and production of artificial human milk, or baby formula, and society's emphasis on the alleged benefits of bottle-feeding. Bottle-feeding enabled mothers to spend more time apart from their babies. With rising affluence in the middle class and an increased value placed on individualism, separate bedrooms for parents and children became more common and culturally fashionable. Family members, childcare experts, and pediatricians stressed the importance of solitary sleep for the child and intimacy for the parents.

By the mid-1900s, it became very common, for the first time in human history, for babies to be bottle-fed and then placed to sleep on their stomachs (to promote uninterrupted sleep) in a room far from the sensory range and supervision of their parents. It did not work out very well for babies. This development gave rise to the epidemic of Sudden Infant Death Syndrome (SIDS). Culture changed, but the human infant's need for breastmilk and contact with the mother's body did not.

I touched on the social values of autonomy and independence earlier, but our desire to raise independent children has led to a false belief that they must be independent from the very beginning of their lives. Parents worry when their infant dislikes sleeping alone or craves their attention. This ignores the fact that infants are, biologically, contact seekers who are—and should be—dependent on parents and caregivers. Yet, in attempts to raise self-reliant children, many parents have decided that it's best for an infant to sleep alone, allowing their ideological beliefs to guide their parenting technique, rather than scientific research or even their instincts.

Parental instinct has also been undermined by Western medical authoritative knowledge. With the rise of science and technology, people began to trust "authorities" and "officials" more than their own instincts. However, current recommendations for infant sleep originated mainly from white men, many of whom never cared for their own infants, and based their conclusions not on empirical scientific research, but on their ideological beliefs. And parents heeded their advice.

Pediatricians and childcare experts erroneously claimed that separate sleep promoted an infant's ability to "self-soothe," and would lead to infants becoming independent children and more satisfied adults. Opponents of cosleeping falsely claim that "problems" are inevitable and that social skills and independence might only be obtained by children through the minimization of parental interventions and contact, supported by solitary sleep. Nothing could be further from the scientific truth.

What we have come to learn in recent decades is that if any developmental differences can be associated with sleeping arrangements, the opposite of common beliefs is true: it is cosleeping children, and not solitary-sleeping children, who appear to be more independent.[31]

Unfortunately, the cultural legacy of independent sleep remains truly ingrained in Western societies, perpetuated by pediatric sleep "experts" whose training took place when most mothers were feeding their babies formula or breastmilk substitutes. But the world has shifted away from formula-feeding. With the majority of mothers now choosing to breastfeed at least some of the time, infants sleeping in separate rooms has become impractical owing to the fact that breastfeeding requires short intervals between feeds.

This historical and cultural context makes it easier to understand why it was assumed that early nighttime infant separation from the parents was necessary to produce happy, confident, emotionally healthy, independent future adults, alongside magnificently energized parents. Without any anthropological or biological studies, which would have cast serious doubt on these assumptions, separate sleep spaces and controlled bottle-feeding were promoted.

And so we arrive at the classic image of a sleeping infant in Western industrialized societies: alone, detached, sucking on a bottle, without any parental contact.

---------- ) ----------

## Cosleeping: The Normal and Safe Way for Mothers and Babies to Sleep

For most of human history (and before written records) covering hundreds of thousands of years, mothers have effectively combined cosleeping and breastfeeding to provide for their babies' immediate social, psychological, and physical needs. Already, you are probably getting the sense that, whether born in Indiana or Papua New Guinea, human infants are strikingly vulnerable and slow developing, and must rely on their parents' touch, carrying, and feeding for survival.

In this immature state, human babies are, for the first few months of life, at least, unable to efficiently regulate their body temperature without a caregiver being in proximity. They are unable to make effective antibodies, which naturally occur in mothers' breastmilk, to protect themselves from bacteria and viruses. Human infants cannot control their bladder or bowels, speak, make tools, digest large molecules, or walk.

Due to this extreme human developmental immaturity, babies require parental (especially maternal) smell, touch, sounds, and movement in order to feel secure and to have their physical needs met. All primate infants, including humans, biologically expect to be in close contact and proximity with their caregivers. In fact, human infants are not adapted to the outside physical environment, but only to what the mother's body offers them.

Cosleeping, traditionally an extension of our human need for infant-parent closeness, is significant to our evolutionary endurance. Anthropological studies that examined the sleeping customs of families in tropical, nonindustrialized cultures have discovered that all of these hunter-gatherer and tribal-level societies share sleep with their babies.[32] Researchers consider these societies to be most similar ecologically and adaptively to prehistoric cultures, whose members coslept in order to ensure the survival and well-being of their infants (and our species).

As we know, separate sleep was made possible with the advent of modern infant care innovations, specifically including artificial milk or cow's milk, prone infant sleep, cribs, and nurseries. However, along with these trends came another alarming development—babies in increasing numbers were not waking up.

Sudden Infant Death Syndrome (SIDS), for which we scientists still have no complete explanation, started to grow. We still do not know the exact causes of SIDS, also known as cot or crib death. We only know that there may be many causes that interact with a range of possible environmental stressors, which we will get into later. SIDS is diagnosed only following a full toxicological report and post-mortem analysis, when all other causes of death have been ruled out. SIDS remains, then, a "diagnosis by exclusion." When SIDS was first defined as a medical entity in 1963, the death rate from this tragic syndrome was between 2–3 babies per 1,000 live births in most Western nations.

> Babies who sleep in their own rooms are sometimes twice as likely to succumb to SIDS.

Researchers now know that placing babies on their stomachs, in the prone position, is the most significant risk factor for SIDS, with maternal smoking (either before or after the baby's birth) coming in at a close second. We see in the data that babies who are fed infant formula die from SIDS, congenital abnormalities, or illness in higher numbers than babies who are breastfed. And we know that babies who sleep in their own rooms are sometimes twice as likely to succumb to SIDS, according to recent studies in Great Britain, New Zealand, and a variety of countries in Western Europe. In many Asian cultures, where cosleeping and breastfeeding (as well as low maternal smoking rates) are the norms, SIDS is either considered rare or is simply unheard of.

Unfortunately, many well-intentioned people, professional and lay alike, believe that all forms of cosleeping are harmful and cannot be made safe. In my opinion, to condemn all forms of cosleeping—without distinguishing between safe and unsafe factors, or considering how benefits and risks vary according to context—is to confuse personal preferences and ideologies with good public policy strategies, and better, less-biased science.

The presumption made by some medical authorities that a mother is not able to respond to her infant's needs while sleeping is refuted by human infant survival throughout history and prehistory. 45–60 million years of primate evolution—the time period within which primate infants slept only in their mother's arms—can't be all wrong. On a more practical level, such a view is refuted by our own extensive laboratory studies,[33] by cross-cultural data on infancy and bedsharing worldwide,[34] and by evolutionary data[35] that have linked mother-infant cosleeping with breastfeeding.

Most importantly, the idea that any and all bedsharing is inherently dangerous is refuted by mothers themselves,[36] who currently sleep safely with their babies, or did so in the recent past. To perpetuate to the public the idea that the mother's body, no matter what her intentions, motives, and capacities, represents an inherent threat to her infant is not only scientifically unsupportable, but far more dangerous in the long run than the idea of cosleeping itself.

I worry more and more about our society's willingness to overlook parental rights, acquired wisdom, and parental judgments in favor of an increasingly impersonal and inappropriate one-size-must-fit-all medical parenting science. Many previous safety recommendations proved to be independent risk factors for

SIDS, which killed tens of thousands of Euro-Western infants. Aside from getting it wrong on a scale with which we are already tragically familiar, such a worldview undermines parents' rights to make informed decisions of their own and to read evidence differently from civil or medical authorities. Even worse, it leads them to doubt their own abilities to assess what their infants really need, preventing them from making their infants happy, safe, and healthy.

# Part 2

The Politically-Charged
Conversations Around
Cosleeping

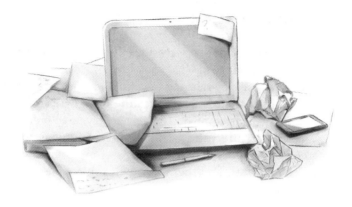

CHAPTER 4

# Controversy, Confusion, and Flawed Conclusions

Cosleeping advice is not readily available from most health professionals. Many individuals and organizations refuse to offer advice even if a parent asks. In fact, lactation specialists and nurses employed by many American and European hospitals are threatened with losing their jobs should they even mention the word cosleeping, let alone give advice on how to reduce risks associated with particular kinds of cosleeping. Many families also feel embarrassed or afraid to ask friends and family for advice, due to the widespread and heavy-handed messaging of anti-bedsharing campaigns.[37]

Public health institutions, including the main authority on infant health and safety, the American Academy of Pediatrics (AAP), believe that bedsharing is a dangerous practice. They claim that all bedsharing invariably increases the risk for Sudden Infant Death Syndrome (SIDS) and nighttime suffocation, and that the only way to solve this problem is to push the anti-bedsharing message. The potentially devastating consequences make conversations about cosleeping particularly delicate; however, the conversations must be had.

A growing number of families are still choosing to bedshare, whether intentionally or out of necessity, but these parents often have little or no knowledge of what constitutes a safe bedsharing environment. Tragically, by refusing to discuss or offer guidelines for safe bedsharing practices, public health officials are actually contributing to the bedsharing deaths they are trying to prevent.

The factors that affect the accuracy and truthfulness of the research used in this "bedsharing debate" are sometimes shockingly complicated, and there are many critical pieces of information that are being overlooked. It is extremely difficult to determine the true risks and benefits associated with bedsharing, but, if we take into account all perspectives and factors, we will be able to make informed decisions about where our babies sleep and how to keep them safe.

———————— ❱ ————————

## What Really Causes SIDS?

I am of the impression that there is currently much less research being devoted to the potential causes of Sudden Infant Death Syndrome (SIDS) than in the '70s and '80s. The majority of attention and funding is now being invested into how to prevent it. This isn't necessarily bad, but it's unfortunate that we're unlikely to find more definitive answers to what biological factors predispose infants to SIDS. Some researchers have hinted that SIDS may be eliminated altogether if environmental risk factors were eradicated, including any and all bedsharing.[38] Maybe this explains why, in recent years, so little headway has been made in understanding what causes SIDS. If we can indeed pinpoint and eliminate the main environmental risks that make SIDS more likely, then so be it, and all the better. The problem is that bedsharing is not actually a risk factor. Rather than eliminating the practice, we need to concentrate on discovering the true specific factors that can make bedsharing dangerous.

Regarding an actual "cause" of SIDS, a leading theory among

scientists is that an infant's failure to arouse from a deep sleep is a major contributing factor. Infants do not have the same self-arousal mechanisms that older children and adults have. It is possible for a baby to fall asleep and not wake up without external stimulation, because his or her body has not yet developed the ability to wake itself. SIDS rates decline greatly at four months of age, as infants begin to develop these arousal capabilities, and decline even more at six months.

Under-developed self-arousal mechanisms are much more likely to be a problem when combined with prematurity and other congenital risk factors—some identified and some not. Researchers have found in SIDS victims evidence of brainstem abnormalities in the neurotransmitters that are responsible for arousal and other autonomic responses. This likely explains why some infants die and some do not when placed in the same sleep environment, and explains why some infants still succumb even when placed in a safe sleep environment.[39]

Known external risk factors for SIDS can also exacerbate underdeveloped arousal capabilities. These risk factors include maternal smoking during pregnancy, formula or cow's milk in place of breastmilk, parental smoking in general, lack of bodily contact and stimulation, prone sleeping (infant lying on his or her stomach), prematurity, overheating, and infants sleeping in a separate room.

Smoking alone is not given the attention it deserves. It should be stressed that safe sleep actually begins before the baby is born, as maternal smoking while pregnant further diminishes an infant's capacity to awaken in order to terminate apneas. A smokeless gestation is the first critical step toward safe infant sleep, followed by initiating breastfeeding postnatally, and maintaining a smoke-free environment for your baby. At least 60% of SIDS occurrences could be eliminated following these three guidelines.

> Safe sleep actually begins before the baby is born.

Failure to arouse can make ordinarily harmless sleeping conditions and positions life threatening, as the infant cannot awake to adjust themselves or cry for help. If these theories are

# How Useful Are Apnea Monitors for Sleep Safety and SIDS Prevention?

Some parents use an infant apnea monitor at home in an attempt to reduce the likelihood of SIDS. Home monitoring has changed significantly since it was introduced over 40 years ago. The machines have improved from a simple alarm system to a sophisticated piece of equipment capable of tracking numerous vital signs. The reasons for using one have also changed. The home monitor was initially used with the belief that it could reduce the incidence of Sudden Infant Death Syndrome (SIDS). However, the American Academy of Pediatrics has taken the stance that monitors are not an effective way to reduce SIDS.[40] My own opinion is that their usefulness is highly limited. While monitors might be of value for selected, potentially ill infants, there is no evidence that their use decreases the incidence of SIDS.[41, 42]

I understand why some parents might feel more secure when using them. However, these monitors can create a false sense of security. While they can be used to help reduce the likelihood that a child will die in his or her sleep, they afford parents no guarantees. The monitors are not always reliable; for example, they cannot detect situations where breathing movements continue but an obstruction in the windpipe prevents oxygen reaching the baby's lungs. The alarm may also be prevented from going off by other body movements unrelated to breathing. False alarms from temperamental monitors have also been an issue. A survey by *Which?* magazine found that seven out of ten mothers had switched the monitor off after repeated false alarms.[43]

In addition, home monitoring can negatively affect parents. Parents using these devices have been shown to have higher stress scores, greater levels of fatigue, and poorer health than parents of infants without monitors.[44] In most cases, cosleeping will be a more effective and comfortable monitoring system. With this in mind, parents should focus on avoiding risk factors and following established safety precautions for preventing SIDS.

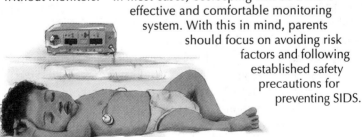

correct, then infants who breastsleep should actually be at the lowest risk of SIDS. Although anecdotal, an internet study of over 200 bedsharing mothers presents, in detail, instances when the parents may have saved their infant's life by bedsharing (see Appendix IV).[36] Many reported that during the night, they noticed that their baby was not breathing and turning blue, or making unusual gurgling or choking sounds, but they were quickly able to intervene and help restart the infant's breathing. Studies by Drs. Blair and Fleming also show that breastleeping with a three-month-old baby may be protective against SIDS, in the absence of hazardous factors.

This should not be surprising; after all, the countries with the highest rates of bedsharing—such as China—also have the lowest rates of SIDS.[45] It should be pointed out that the majority of these babies breastsleep with non-smoking mothers. The positive association between bedsharing and reduced SIDS was unintentionally confirmed in an international study in 2000.[34] In this study, as bedsharing rates generally rose, region by region and city by city, Sudden Infant Death Sydrome rates generally declined. Researchers called this finding a "paradox." The lead authors were committed to the idea that wherever bedsharing rates are high, SIDS rates must be high, too. They were confused and surprised to find that the opposite was true. Interestingly, their explanation for the "paradox" is exactly what I have been arguing for years: that bedsharing rates can lead to positive, if not protective, outcomes when practiced safely in the context of breastfeeding.

So, why does breastsleeping make it easier for babies to arouse from sleep? There are a few reasons, which I will describe in greater detail later on (see Chapter 6). All-night laboratory studies demonstrate that more maternal inspections, more infant arousals, and less deep sleep among infants occur when mothers and infants sleep together routinely.[46] Basically, when sleeping in close proximity, the parents' small movements and vocalizations help the baby stay in a lighter phase of sleep, and allow the infant to wake more frequently. I call these brief awakenings partner-induced arousals—when one of the sleepers causes the other to arouse, like the baby momentarily opening his or her eyes after the mother coughs or sneezes. The smells of mother's breastmilk and other sensory exchanges also prevent infants from spending too much time in deep sleep, for which they are not always prepared.

This positive effect of breastsleeping also applies to other forms of cosleeping; three studies in Scotland, New Zealand, and England concluded that there is a significantly decreased SIDS risk when the infant is roomsharing, as opposed to sleeping alone.

Breastfeeding and cosleeping are behaviorally, biologically, and functionally inter-connected, which is why we argue that breastsleeping (i.e., bedsharing in the context of breastfeeding) in particular should not be equated with the risks associated with other forms of bedsharing. Certainly it is much safer than bedsharing with a bottle- or formula-fed infant. The sensory experiences, sleep architecture, maternal vigilance, and mutual arousals experienced by breastfeeding mother-baby pairs converge to potentially reduce SIDS.

Breastsleeping allows for regular inspections and physiological regulation of the baby, as our laboratory studies and others have shown.[47] A breastfeeding mother typically rouses if the baby stops breathing or moves into a risky position, or if blankets cover the baby's head. All studies confirm that breastsleeping also increases milk production and breastfeeding frequency, better equipping babies with a larger quantity of breastmilk containing the nutrition they need, which is known to enhance protection against SIDS.[16, 48] Increased frequency of breastfeeding also means mother and baby are waking throughout the night for feeding opportunities, which again helps the infant remain in a light stage of sleep and provides more practice waking to develop the infant's arousal mechanisms.

You may be thinking, *I thought I wanted to wake up less often, not more!*, but in fact, the concept of sleeping through the night is an unrealistic expectation. It is a very recent Western cultural invention that is not promoted in non-Western cultures. The whole idea that babies need to be "sleep trained" early in life for developmental reasons is a myth—a social construct that threatens healthy breastfeeding and infant brain development (see Chapter 10). In the first year of life, infants should be waking several times throughout the night to breastfeed.

What we call consolidated infant sleep may be convenient for parents, but it does nothing good for babies. While it may be closer to an appropriate sleep model for formula-fed babies, the majority of babies now start off breastfeeding thanks to current pediatric recommendations. This means that the whole concept of sleeping through the night has become obsolete—and worse, has become a barrier to optimal breastfeeding. It is time for this outdated expectation to be (pardon the expression) put to rest!

But, not to fear, this is not bad news for your own sleep schedule; multiple studies show that breastsleeping and roomsharing families actually get equal or more sleep than families who practice solitary sleep. You and your baby may be waking up more often, but these awakenings are briefer and calmer than the disruptions that occur when the baby is placed in another room.

---

## One Message to Curb Two Kinds of Infant Death

If you learn anything from this book, I want it to be that Sudden Infant Death Syndrome (SIDS) is not normally, if at all, caused by a baby sleeping in the same bed with his or her mother, especially a breastfeeding mother, in the absence of other risk factors. In the same way that a baby who dies of SIDS in a crib is not a victim of the crib itself, an infant who dies while bedsharing cannot be said to have died simply because of their location in an adult bed, although this is typically the cited cause.

During the '70s and '80s, before the Back to Sleep® campaign in the '90s, SIDS rates (i.e., crib death) were twice as high as they are now. Babies were being placed in cribs on their stomachs, in rooms by themselves, separated from parental supervision. If the babies were being fed anything but breastmilk, this already totals three independent risk factors for SIDS. However, it is well understood that it wasn't the cribs that were responsible for the deaths, but rather the circumstances within which the crib was being used.

Enter the double standard.

It is unfortunate that, as a consequence of strong historic bias, bedsharing deaths are not handled as objectively or with the same nuance as crib deaths. It should be noted that bedsharing has never been analyzed or studied on a level scientific playing field, which affects the way medical and civil authorities assess the "causes," the "diagnoses," and the "solutions" to infant deaths that occur in adult beds. In our society, bedsharing is deemed, de facto, an "unsafe sleep space." No matter what independent risk factors were involved or were not involved in a bedsharing infant's death, it is presumed to be a SUID (Sudden Unexpected Infant Death). This umbrella term encompasses both SIDS and suffocation cases (SASS, or Sleep Associated Suffocation and Strangulation), but the term generally connotes a suffocation case.

Let me illustrate it this way: if a baby dies sleeping on his or her stomach in an adult bed, the cause of death is said to be bedsharing. The diagnosis *should* be that of a SIDS death, but it is instead called a SUID—a potential suffocation owing to the death occurring in an adult bed. The fact that the baby was sleeping on his or her stomach, which is an obvious risk factor for SIDS, is not thought to be the reason the infant died, although it would have been considered the cause of death had that same infant died sleeping this way in a crib. A recent paper reported that in 82% of alleged suffocation deaths, the infants were found sleeping on their stomachs.[49]

In cases where there are other risk factors present, such as the parents being desensitized by drugs or alcohol, these might be similarly ignored, and the cause of death, unrelated to the infant's location in an adult bed, would still be attributed to bedsharing. This system exaggerates the risk of SUID or SASS in bedsharing situations, serving to further build a case against bedsharing, while ignoring those factors that actually cause the deaths.

Dr. Peter S. Blair, a prominent SIDS researcher from the United Kingdom and good friend of mine, recently conversed with U.S. medical examiners in a meeting at Harvard University. He found that physicians have been told over and over that bedsharing is a dangerous practice. Medical examiners are reluctant to use the term SIDS for deaths that occur in an unsafe sleep environment, which currently includes bedsharing, regardless of other relevant circumstances. In Dr. Blair's words, "they want to red flag bedsharing, which is fine from an epidemiological perspective (to monitor associated risk factors) but should play no part in causal classification unless much more detailed evidence is available."[50]

Instead of SIDS, a medical examiner will write on the death certificate something like, *undetermined possible asphyxia given that the infant was bedsharing*. Dr. Blair says that when this happens, the

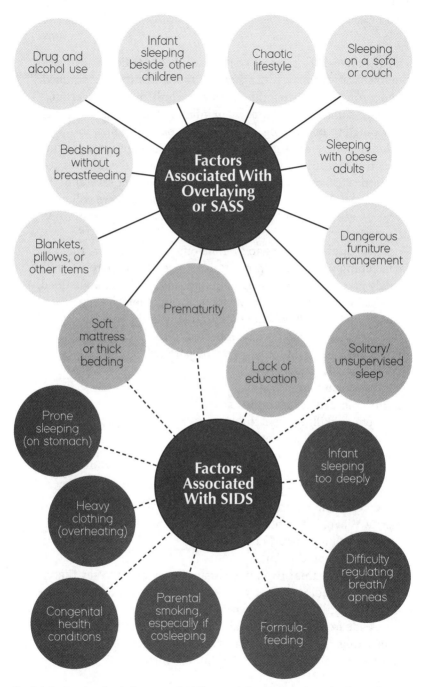

*Fig. 2.1 Cosleeping deaths have mostly different risk factors from SIDS deaths, and some SIDS risks (like heavy sleeping or inability to terminate apneas) are reduced by breastsleeping. However, cosleeping families must be aware that some SIDS risk are potentially exacerbated by bedsharing, such as parental smoking or overheating from heavy clothes.*

algorithm used by medical systems to categorize deaths will pick up the word "asphyxia." This overrides the word "undetermined," and wrongly classifies the death as a confirmed suffocation without sufficient evidence, again inflating the number of deaths attributed to bedsharing. Dr. Blair and colleagues plan to solve this categorization problem in the next version of the algorithm, but in the meantime have agreed across several countries to monitor SIDS more accurately by merging together several of the categories. "When we do this, the rates in the U.K. are still falling year by year," says Dr. Blair, "but in the U.S. they seem to be flat-lining."[50]

Too often, coroners and public officials will report that all cosleeping deaths are "preventable," even if the parents are safely practicing breastsleeping. I find this cruel and unjustified, especially in cases without any forensic or pathological postmortem study. It is entirely possible for an infant to die in an adult bed due to reasons that are not connected to the sleep location, and could not have been foreseen by the parents. Parents deserve a comprehensive, nuanced, and compassionate investigation, not unfounded accusations of accidentally killing their child.

Public health officials will also tell parents that cosleeping in general increases the risk of SIDS, which isn't true. This statement suffers from a lack of clarity. What kind of cosleeping are they talking about, and what exactly do they mean when they say this? Even if we assume they mean to say that bedsharing, not general cosleeping, increases SIDS risks, the statement still cannot be proven.

> Public health officials will tell parents that cosleeping in general increases SIDS risks, which isn't true.

Aside from parental smoking or possible overheating while bedsharing, the physical dangers associated with bedsharing are not necessarily related to SIDS, but are instead risk factors for SASS.

It is important to understand that SIDS and SASS are two separate kinds of infant death with different associated risks. When following proper safety precautions, avoiding

SASS risk factors, and breastfeeding their infant, parents can all but eliminate the chance of suffocation or overlaying while bedsharing. Moreover, merely having an infant sleeping in a room with a committed adult caregiver (any kind of cosleeping) actually reduces the chance of an infant dying from SIDS or from an accident by one half.[42]

However, cosleeping in the form of bedsharing, including breastsleeping, is definitely more complex and less stable than crib sleeping. There are situations that would make deciding to bedshare a bad choice, introducing risk factors for both SASS and SIDS. These include an improper sleep environment (sleeping on a couch, recliner, chair, or waterbed), sleeping with fluffy or loose blankets around the baby, placing a baby to sleep on a pillow, having multiple children in the bed, keeping stuffed animals in the bed, or pushing the bed against a wall where a baby could slip into a gap and suffocate. Bedsharing should not occur if either parent is a smoker, if either parent is under the influence of drugs or alcohol, or if the mother smoked during her pregnancy. Read more about avoiding risk factors in Part 4.

No sleeping arrangement guarantees full protection. It is still possible for an occasional suffocation to occur in any situation, despite careful precautions. For example, over a quarter of suffocation deaths in the U.S. occur in a crib.[49] However, to operate under the assumption that if a suffocation can happen then it will, or that this sort of tragedy is highly likely to happen, is a misguided way of thinking that I have been arguing against for many years.

In any case, whether involving cribs or adult beds, risky sleep practices leading to infant deaths are more likely to occur when parents lack access to comprehensive safety information. This flow of information is blocked because parents are judged to be incapable of maintaining a safe bedsharing environment, so public health messages simply warn, *just never do it*. Such recommendations misrepresent the true function and significance of bedsharing, the importance of breastfeeding, and the critical extent to which dangerous practices can be modified. From a biological perspective, mother-infant cosleeping in a safe environment can contribute significantly to infant and maternal health and well-being, and has very likely saved infant lives by protecting against SIDS. Don't forget that it's much easier to quantify the occurrence of infant deaths than it is to count the number of times a mother's presence has prevented the cascade of physiological events necessary for SIDS to occur.

———————— ❱ ————————

## Complications of Collecting and Analyzing Statistics

The American Academy of Pediatrics (AAP) released papers in 2005, 2011, and 2014 labeling any and all bedsharing as "hazardous." Before their first paper was published, I was invited by Dr. John Kattwinkel, then-chair of the Infant Sleep Position and SIDS Subcommittee, to participate as an ad hoc advisor.

I submitted a "White Paper" sharing my research data on the behavior and physiology of bedsharing, contributing a much-needed point of view. However, the research I provided was not reflected in the published recommendations. Input from the Breastfeeding Subcommittee of the AAP, at the time headed by Dr. Larry Gartner, was also ignored. The Breastfeeding Subcommittee, in contrast to the SIDS subcommittee, supported breastfeeding mothers' rights to bedshare and to find support from health professionals. I worked with the breastfeeding group during this time, and we mistakenly thought some kind of compromise between the two committees would take place. It didn't.

It is important to know that the case against bedsharing has been based exclusively on population-wide, epidemiological studies—meaning broadly-based studies on the causes, distribution, and possible prevention of sleep-related infant deaths. Essentially, these are statistical evaluations of degrees of risks associated with crib sleeping versus bedsharing. A handful of recent studies have investigated the risks of other sleep environments, but the main question still centers around how many babies sleep in cribs and survive, compared to how many babies sleep in bed with their parents (or other adults) and survive.

This comparison seems pretty simple. However, statistics are only as valid as the careful choice and defining of variables, the accuracy and completeness of the data collected, the kinds of questions asked or not asked, and the interpretation of the data by investigators. Herein lies one of the problems inherent in many scientific explorations, particularly in studies conducted on this issue. Additionally, epidemiologists only cover one of many lines of pertinent SIDS research. Other, equally relevant lines of research have not been taken into consideration.

It is here where the principles of Evidence-Based Medicine (EBM), fundamental to the formulation of public health recommendations, have been violated. The process advocated for by the primary architects of EBM requires health recommendations to be based on comprehensive studies that are clear about their limitations. Dr. David Sackett, the original authority on EBM, also warns specifically against translating findings from large epidemiological studies (such as the country-wide SIDS studies) into broad public health recommendations without properly testing the hypotheses made from the data. This is fundamental to the field of epidemiology in general, as it allows us to understand how and why a practice is consistently a risk or not, and how environmental factors modify those risks. This topic will be further explored in Chapter 5.

> Public health recommendations fail to reflect that bedsharing safety cannot be quantified in any simple way, or determined solely by location.

Statistical decisions, research practices, and the creation of public health recommendations are treated with shocking laxity when it comes to cosleeping and bedsharing. While all of the studies separate out various "co-factors," like infant sleep position and feeding method, not all studies define the variables in the same way. Often, such key relevant co-factors are missing altogether, and the data must be inferred from patterns in other data, using statistical algorithms. The most commonly missing data happens to be critical, and that is whether or not drugs and alcohol were involved in each case. This information is essential to know when assessing how any given bedsharing baby died.

While attention is paid to these co-factors in scientific papers, public health recommendations fail to reflect that bedsharing safety cannot be quantified in any simple way, or determined solely by location. This is because so many critical social, physical, and even psychological factors matter, and make all the difference in our ability to understand bedsharing outcomes. I have always said that we should never underestimate factors such as how much parents know about bedsharing safety and how much the practice means to them.

Especially in the earlier epidemiological studies conducted throughout Ireland, Scotland, Australia, New Zealand, and most of Europe, there was little consistency between and within studies. All variations of cosleeping were being lumped together and called different things. Dr. Helen Ball, an infant sleep expert in the U.K., states that, in many epidemiological studies, "Data were not comparable between studies or even between cases and controls in the same study,"[51] making it impossible to draw meaningful conclusions about what does or does not increase the risk of SUID in a bedsharing situation. For example, the term "adult bed" often included dangerous sofas, sofa chairs, recliners, makeshift beds, and waterbeds—which are known to be unsafe cosleeping environments, but account for a large portion of the reported bedsharing deaths.

One prominent study published in the journal *Pediatrics* was conducted on a U.S. population of poor, high-risk mothers and infants living in Cleveland. Instances involving obese women sleeping on couches with their babies were counted in the final analysis as "bedsharing deaths." The authors concluded that, to err on the side of caution, bedsharing should be avoided. The problem is that the study wasn't about bedsharing at all; it was about sofa or couch sleeping, under questionable and very dangerous circumstances. The extra risk factors were ignored when determining why the infant actually died. Other studies included occurrences where the infant had been sleeping with a parent at some point during the night—or even in the last two weeks—but had actually died in a crib![52]

The other major problem, rarely mentioned by anyone, is how to best collect truthful and accurate data on how many parents are actually bedsharing. This is an especially difficult problem in Western industrialized societies, which have historically privileged the practice of solitary infant sleep. In the past, solitary sleep has been described as both normal and healthy, as well as desirable—including the early consolidation of infant sleep (i.e., sleeping through the night).

> Parents have admitted that they are more likely to report where they are told their baby is supposed to sleep—which is in a crib—rather than where they actually sleep.

Bedsharing studies significantly undercount how many babies have bedshared and survived, in comparison to the number of infants who bedshared and died. This is a critical data set because parents falsely reporting that they did not bedshare (when they actually did, and their babies survived) artificially inflates the proportion of deaths occurring in adult beds.

Thus far, no epidemiological study that I know of has pre-tested how parents were interpreting and responding to questions

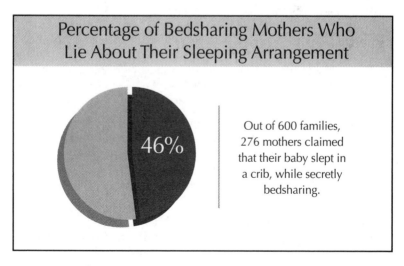

## Percentage of Bedsharing Mothers Who Lie About Their Sleeping Arrangement

46%

Out of 600 families, 276 mothers claimed that their baby slept in a crib, while secretly bedsharing.

*Fig. 2.2 A poll in Great Britain, commissioned by Sarah Ockwell-Smith of the website Gentle Parenting, revealed that 46% of parents had not told their healthcare providers they were bedsharing, for fear of being judged.*[53]

about where their baby sleeps. Judging from other lines of research by Drs. Helen Ball and Kathleen Kendall-Tackett, parents are purposefully or inadvertently not revealing to researchers their true bedsharing practices. Many parents, by their own reports,[36, 37] fear reprisal or criticism—or worse, having their children taken away—if they report that they bedshare. Dr. Ball would have missed 40% of families that bedshared in Great Britain had she

# Is It Bad to Lie to My Healthcare Provider About Bedsharing With My Baby?

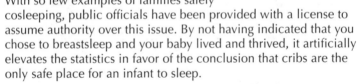

You should always be honest with your healthcare provider in general, but it is especially timely that bedsharing parents be upfront about their sleeping arrangements so it can be accurately documented. By lying, the science of bedsharing becomes very skewed. With so few examples of families safely cosleeping, public officials have been provided with a license to assume authority over this issue. By not having indicated that you chose to breastsleep and your baby lived and thrived, it artificially elevates the statistics in favor of the conclusion that cribs are the only safe place for an infant to sleep.

If you tell your healthcare provider that you are bedsharing, you will likely be told that you are putting your baby at risk. Hearing this from a person you trust can be heartbreaking. However, if you are carefully following safe breastsleeping practices, we know this statement is untrue. Use the opportunity to educate them as to why and how you are bedsharing, and, at the very least, get a conversation going.

Also, keep in mind that lying about bedsharing inadvertently supports the idea that something is wrong with it. You may have to listen to a quick lecture, but telling your healthcare provider the truth can legitimize breastsleeping for you and your fellow bedsharing parents.

not either filmed the behavior in her subjects' homes or probed more deeply into their responses to questions about where their baby sleeps.[54]

This problem is more relevant in the United States, where the issue of bedsharing has only been presented in an extremely negative light, with bedsharing parents often demonized in the media. The issue is framed in terms of whether to practice it or not, with nothing in between. As we know, the answer given by U.S. authorities is *just never do it*. While most babies sleep in more than one place during the night, parents have admitted that they are more likely to report where they are told their baby is supposed to sleep—which is in a crib—rather than where they actually sleep. When asked, many parents who claim their infant sleeps in a crib leave out the fact that the baby only starts the night in the crib and is relocated to the parents' bed upon the first feed, or upon the infant crying in the middle of the night.

It has to be stressed that reported bedsharing numbers are affected by the ferocity with which medical and civil authorities have attacked and threatened bedsharing families. In some communities, public health professionals have threatened to declare adults who bedshare to be "unfit parents." The contempt shown by some health professionals and those involved in the judicial process inhibits parents' willingness to admit their bedsharing behavior to anyone, including their own family members.

———————— ❯ ————————

# Interpreting Research Regarding Bedsharing Risk: A Conversation With Epidemiologist Dr. Peter Blair

I have had the good fortune and privilege to be both a friend, colleague, and collaborator with Dr. Peter Blair, whom I first met through his mentor, Dr. Peter Fleming. I am lucky to say that Dr. Fleming is also one of my collaborators and good friends, and is a world class researcher—awarded by the Queen of Great Britain herself for his pioneering SIDS research. In the early

'90s, after the publication of my SIDS monograph in 1986, I was invited by Dr. Fleming to his laboratory in St. Michaels Hospital at Bristol University. I was asked to present my evolutionary-based hypothesis on how solitary sleep and formula-feeding contribute to SIDS. This is where I met Dr. Blair, who has become one of the world's premier SIDS researchers and epidemiologists.

As an epidemiologist, Dr. Blair has firsthand experience gathering and analyzing data on the causes and distribution of sleep-related deaths. For this reason, he is the best person to help us decipher what epidemiological studies, with all of their pitfalls, actually say about the risks associated with bedsharing. We are going to explore his important insights and experiences here. The section below is what Dr. Blair shared with me, and I am privileged to be able to use his words to make sure I get everything right!

According to Dr. Blair, prior to the Back to Sleep® campaigns in the 1990s, the evidence tying bedsharing to SIDS was mixed. Following the campaigns, we witnessed a dramatic fall in SIDS deaths overall; however, it appeared that the risk of bedsharing death increased among mothers who smoked during or after their pregnancies. Studies also pointed to a significantly increased risk of danger when parents consumed alcohol or drugs prior to bedsharing. Additionally, high risks appeared when parents slept on sofas and chairs. But, in these studies, the risk of bedsharing incidents among non-smokers who slept in a normal adult bed appeared negligible.[55]

Both Drs. Blair and Fleming initially interpreted these findings as possibly being something unique to the English and Irish populations until they examined the U.S. data. Information from 24 states between 2004 and 2012 showed, as Dr. Blair reports, 889 sofa deaths with a parent on the same surface. A quarter of these were classified as SIDS and the rest as either "ill-defined" or as SASS deaths (technically called ASSB; see the Glossary for more information).

It is at this point that Dr. Blair began to wonder whether or not there were actually SIDS risks associated with bedsharing in the absence of hazardous factors. To answer this, Dr. Blair, Dr. Fleming, and their research team, along with researchers who directed epidemiological studies in other countries, looked to data from studies that focused more specifically on hazardous environments. This led to two different pooled analyses, one led by Dr. Bob Carpenter,[56] and another by Dr. Blair.[57] The analyses reached opposite conclusions.

Dr. Carpenter found an increased risk of SIDS associated with bedsharing even in the absence of any hazardous factors, while Drs. Blair and Fleming found no risk in the absence of hazardous factors. Creating further confusion, Dr. Blair's research team also found, for the first time, a positive, protective effect against SIDS when bedsharing with babies three months of age or older.

Because of this divergence, the papers were reviewed by Dr. Robert Platt, an independent statistician commissioned by the AAP. Dr. Platt presented his findings at an international SIDS conference in Uruguay in 2016 that Dr. Blair had helped organize. Platt's review found in the studies what is called "attendant bias," a weakness afflicting all observational studies. His main conclusion was that these two studies were basically saying the same thing. How is that possible, and what could explain these conflicting results?

Dr. Blair and Dr. Fleming, and many other researchers, had serious reservations about the Carpenter analysis. They questioned the assumptions made and the manner in which missing data from whole studies was "imputed." This means that the data was statistically constructed through complex calculations or algorithms. Imputing data is usually done for factors collected within a study, not for whole studies that did not include the factor to begin with. The claim that there was a significant risk of SIDS associated with bedsharing among non-smoking, breastfeeding mothers was only found by using imputed data. Since it is inferred instead of collected, imputed data can easily be wrong.

For Dr. Carpenter's analysis, this problem was compounded by the fact that as much as 60% of the data was, in fact, imputed. While imputation can be appropriate when information on co-factors is missing, Dr. Blair emphasizes that it is definitely pushing the boundaries when the study results depend on a significant number of missing variables that need to be constructed.

Primarily, what was missing from the analysis were questions about alcohol consumption and drug use, which we know are extremely important factors affecting bedsharing safety. These factors, in particular, are based on rates that can vary from study to study or culture to culture, making the validity of the imputed data—and therefore the validity of Dr. Carpenter's analysis and conclusions—suspect.

In contrast, Dr. Blair's analysis had all of the actual data for each of the studies they used, including data on parental alcohol consumption, and they did not have to conduct any imputation calculations. But this wasn't Dr. Blair's main concern with the other analysis. In reading Dr. Carpenter's paper, Dr. Blair saw that the research team found an adjusted risk of 5.1, meaning that bedsharing, even without extra hazards, incurs about five times the risk of dying compared with crib sleeping. But they qualify this alarming statistic by saying these adjusted risk ratios compared bedsharing to a situation where "no other risk factors are present and the baseline risk group is breastfed baby girls placed on their back for sleep by the bed of non-smoking parents having no other risk factors."

> While there is a significant risk associated with bedsharing and maternal smoking, bedsharing was not a significant SUID risk among non-smokers.

Dr. Blair points out that Dr. Carpenter's calculation of an adjusted risk is made against "an idealized reference group where ANY risk factor would obviously be inflated." Bedsharing was being compared to an extremely low-risk group rather than a group representing the population norms. In other words, Dr. Carpenter did not quantify this risk using the normally recognized reference groups of non-bedsharers. Dr. Blair followed this up by saying, "We could do this with our own data, and not just for bedsharing, but it would be impossible to interpret its meaning."[50]

Using an idealized reference group, Dr. Blair maintains, the researcher can't distinguish between what is actually increased risk, coming from the practice of bedsharing, and what is perceived increased risk, coming from a relatively wider gap between the bedsharing risk and an exceptionally low baseline risk.

In his own paper, Dr. Blair's research team did not find a significant risk "even when we limited it to the younger infants and adjusted for other factors in the model." Thus, Dr. Blair's research paper is the only study to date that has truly quantified the SIDS risk associated with bedsharing in the absence of hazards. The risk they arrived at is around 1.0, which essentially means bedsharing is not really a risk, but not really protective either. The risk associated with bedsharing among smokers, however, was four times that of nonsmokers. With alcohol or sofas involved, the risk multiplies by 18, a magnitude higher than any other SIDS risk factor.

Another epidemiological study was recently published by Dr. Ed Mitchell in the *New Zealand Medical Journal*. Dr. Blair reflects, "I have read it, and my understanding is that they did not seem to ask about alcohol consumption (perhaps because it was culturally sensitive), but found a significant interaction between bedsharing and maternal smoking."[50] This means that the combination of bedsharing and maternal smoking leads to a greatly increased risk of SUID. They also found that, while there is a significant risk associated with bedsharing and maternal smoking, bedsharing was not a significant SUID risk among non-smokers, which is consistent with Dr. Blair's study.

Regardless of the statistical problems associated with bedsharing data, adult beds do need to be made safe, and precautions do need to be taken to remove risk factors for SIDS and SASS (see Part 4) in bedsharing environments. For babies younger than three months who do not breastfeed, there may (inconclusively) be an increased risk of danger, though it is not comparable to some of the other risks posed by smoking and drinking alcohol.

However, what about situations where parents don't drink or smoke? What about babies who are breastfed and are not premature or underweight?

The relative risk of death for full-term, normal-weight infants who sleep in a safely-configured bed with a breastfeeding mother is far smaller than that of infants who sleep in a crib in another room. For babies older than three months of age, there is no detectable increased risk of SIDS among families that practice bedsharing in the absence of other hazards.[17, 56]

This can be clearly seen in the data on bedsharing deaths

reported among primarily indigenous Alaskans. The Alaska Division of Public Health policies differs from the AAP's recommendations, having publicly stated that "infants may safely share a bed for sleeping if this occurs with a nonsmoking, unimpaired caregiver on a standard, adult, non-water mattress." Many Alaskan mothers report frequent bedsharing under these safe conditions.

Drs. Margaret Blabey and Bradford D. Gessner examined 13 years of Alaskan infant deaths that occurred while bedsharing "to assess the contribution of known risk factors." As explained in their paper, they "examined vital records, medical records, autopsy reports, and first responder reports" for most infant deaths between 1992 and 2004. About 13% of deaths (126 infants) occurred while bedsharing, but 99% of these had at least one modifiable risk factor present, including maternal tobacco or marijuana use, sleeping with an impaired person, and infants sleeping prone. In other words "almost all bedsharing deaths occurred in association with multiple risk factors…; this suggests that bedsharing alone does not increase the risk of infant death."[58] If modifiable factors were eliminated, and especially if breastfeeding were involved, I would predict that breastsleeping will prove to be the safest way to bedshare.

———— ❯ ————

## Bedsharing Deaths, Structural Racism, and Poverty

There is no doubt that black Americans face more stressors in their daily lives, in general, than many other racial groups. This is not just because they have less control over and access to financial resources, due to generations of inequality, but also because of the constant structural, social, and psychological violence of racism and general discrimination.

SUID rates generally parallel increases in degrees of racism, poverty, and marginalization, especially in urban locales and amongst indigenous peoples like Native Americans. However, these effects are not felt equally across minority groups. Because indigenous peoples and black Americans, in particular, face more severe socio-cultural and economic marginalization, almost all studies show negative impacts on the health and well-being of people in these groups. This includes significant increases in infant illness and mortality before issues of sleeping arrangements are even considered.

A survey in a 2005 issue of *Pediatrics* found that the prevalence of bedsharing among black children was five times that of white children in the U.S. While black families top the bedsharing charts, Asian and Hispanic households also report higher rates of bedsharing than white households.[59] Although black American families experience higher-than-average SUID and SIDS rates, Asian and Hispanic households experience lower-than-average SUID and SIDS rates, meaning that bedsharing is not the deciding issue.

Local media stories about bedsharing deaths rarely, if ever, probe into the larger social context. This context includes the high percentage of black babies born prematurely (a risk factor for SIDS) and the existence of other risk factors that are almost always associated with bedsharing deaths in these communities. For

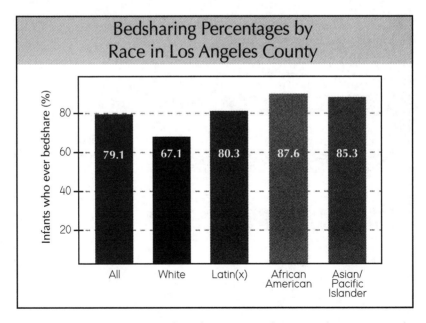

*Fig. 2.3 These percentages come from the responses of 6,246 mothers in Los Angeles County, gathered by the Los Angeles Mommy and Baby (LAMB) Project in 2007.*

example, in the U.S., black mothers initiate breastfeeding at about a 20% lower rate than white mothers. Yet again, before sleeping arrangement even comes into the picture, these babies are at an increased risk of dying. For poor black families living in large cities such as Chicago, Cleveland, the District of Columbia, and St. Louis, the impact of these risk factors is even more pronounced. It is not surprising that where black Americans live in the greatest poverty, the highest numbers of infant deaths attributed to bedsharing take place.[48, 58]

Low breastfeeding rates, in particular, contribute significantly to the likelihood of infant death. A study published by Dr. Renata Forste[60] found that breastfeeding accounts for racial differences in infant mortality "at least as well as low birth weight does." She and her colleagues write: "Breastfed infants are 80% less likely to die before [one year of age] than those who never breastfed,

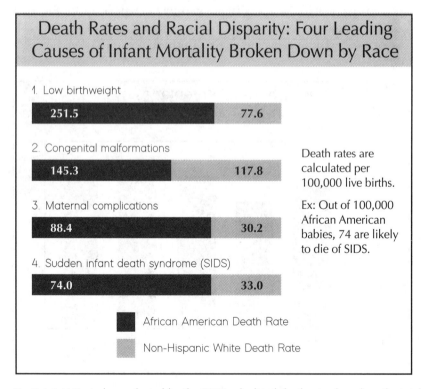

Fig. 2.4 A U.S. study conducted by the CDC calculated death rates based on the total number of infants born and the total number of infant deaths that occured in 2014.

even controlling for low birthweight," and, "For every 100 deaths in the formula-fed group, there were 20 deaths in the breastfed group...the formula group with 100 deaths had five times as many deaths, or a 500% increase in mortality." This is truly an extraordinary statistic that calls on local and national health institutions to lead campaigns promoting breastfeeding, especially in black communities, as stridently as they have driven the anti-bedsharing campaign.

Research has shown that there is a link between living in poverty and high rates of infant deaths. These deaths are not just due to the risks of formula-feeding, but also due to other contextual factors, including other children sleeping next to the infant, bedsharing in a small or cramped bed, the bed being placed close to a wall or furniture where a baby can get stuck, sleeping with an unrelated adult male partner in the bed, and low birthweight. All of these amount to a less stable and safe sleep environment. Unfortunately, medical and civil authorities have not been willing to tackle the social reasons why negative outcomes are associated with bedsharing in these populations or why SIDS rates can be predicted by zip code. Poorer communities have a disproportionate number of bedsharing deaths compared to white and other sub-groups practicing the same sleeping arrangement.

Keep in mind that there is a significant difference between elective and chaotic bedsharing. Elective bedsharing, what I am recommending and advocating for, is when parents make an informed decision to bedshare for the purpose of nurturing and breastfeeding, and are knowledgeable about the risk factors and how to avoid them. In this scenario, we can expect that bedsharing will reduce the risk of SIDS.

Chaotic bedsharing, on the other hand, is when bedsharing is practiced out of necessity rather than as an intentional parenting technique. In this case, parents sleep with their infants because they feel they have no choice due to circumstances like a lack of beds or cribs in the house, the presence of rodents, or numerous other factors. Families who practice chaotic bedsharing also tend to be less knowledgeable of SIDS or SASS risk factors, such as smoking, drugs, alcohol, unsafe beds, or having other children in the bed with an infant.

Unfortunately, poverty and its associated stressors are more likely to cause families living under these conditions to practice chaotic bedsharing, leading to relatively higher numbers of bedsharing deaths compared to elective bedsharing families (typically from higher socioeconomic groups). It's a sad fact that socioeconomic struggles can affect the safety of your child as he or she sleeps, but that is not to say that the environment can't be made safe for lower socioeconomic families through proper education and recommendations from healthcare providers.

For the healthcare providers in question, when choosing to support or not support a family's sleeping arrangement, it's important that the family's intentions and general circumstances are considered. In many cases, the problem is not bedsharing,

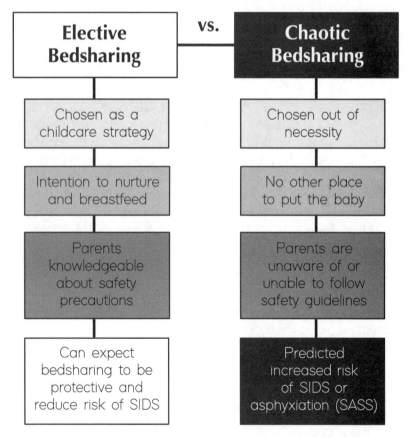

*Fig. 2.5 The differences between elective bedsharing and chaotic bedsharing are illustrated above. Chaotic bedsharing is most often the case for families in low socioeconomic groups, and is much more likely to result in SUID.*

but rather the manner in which it is practiced.

Again, I have to stress that it is a tragedy that such disparities exist between and within groups of people living in the same country, whether it is bedsharing, prematurity, or the birth of underweight infants that accounts for up to 40% of black births. However, using statistics derived from families in low socioeconomic situations to make conclusions about all bedsharing is inappropriate. Instead, this data points to the need to address the perils afflicting poor households directly. This may include simply working harder to share the critical importance of breastfeeding during prenatal care visits with pregnant black mothers. For many reasons that we will explore in Chapter 6, simply choosing to breastfeed greatly increases the safety of bedsharing, reducing risk of injury or suffocation.[34]

———————— ❱ ————————

## Bedsharing Risks in the Larger Perspective

In May of 2018, Michaeleen Doucleff from National Public Radio (NPR) interviewed me about breastsleeping. The question she concentrated on was: *Are doctors exaggerating the risks associated with bedsharing?*

There is no question that same-surface cosleeping can increase the risk of death for an infant, especially where smoking and other safety hazards are present. Doucleff and her colleagues gave us permission to share the graphic on the next page, originally posted on the NPR website, which places into perspective the odds of a baby (or any of us) dying in various situations.

You can see in the chart on the next page that they found the chances of a "low-risk" baby dying in the parents' bed to be about 1 in 16,000, while the chances of an infant dying in a crib next to the parents' bed would be about 1 in 48,000. A low-risk baby is considered a healthy, full-term infant living in a stable, non-smoking home. What isn't calculated in these odds is whether the imaginary baby and mother were bedsharing in the context of breastfeeding. Based on data on the death rates of formula-fed

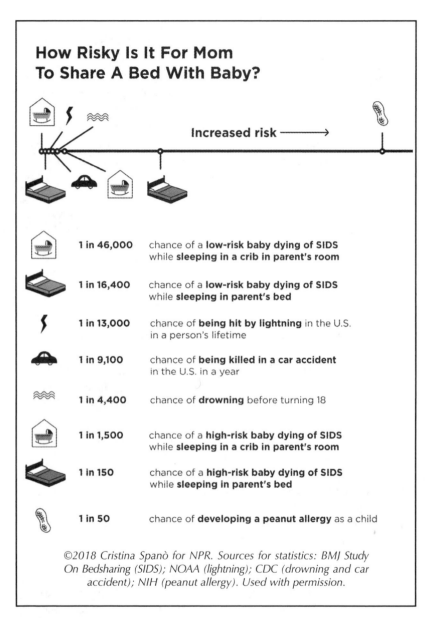

# How Risky Is It For Mom To Share A Bed With Baby?

**Increased risk ⟶**

| | | |
|---|---|---|
| **1 in 46,000** | chance of a **low-risk baby dying of SIDS** while **sleeping in a crib in parent's room** |
| **1 in 16,400** | chance of a **low-risk baby dying of SIDS** while **sleeping in parent's bed** |
| **1 in 13,000** | chance of **being hit by lightning** in the U.S. in a person's lifetime |
| **1 in 9,100** | chance of **being killed in a car accident** in the U.S. in a year |
| **1 in 4,400** | chance of **drowning** before turning 18 |
| **1 in 1,500** | chance of a **high-risk baby dying of SIDS** while **sleeping in a crib in parent's room** |
| **1 in 150** | chance of a **high-risk baby dying of SIDS** while **sleeping in parent's bed** |
| **1 in 50** | chance of **developing a peanut allergy** as a child |

*©2018 Cristina Spanò for NPR. Sources for statistics: BMJ Study On Bedsharing (SIDS); NOAA (lightning); CDC (drowning and car accident); NIH (peanut allergy). Used with permission.*

*Fig. 2.6 SIDS risk is calculated for a 2-month-old female baby of European ancestry. The low-risk baby is of average birth weight and has a 30-year-old mother who does not smoke or drink. The high-risk baby is of low birth weight and has parents who smoke and a 21-year-old mother who has more than two alcoholic drinks regulary.*

versus breastfed infants, it is likely that this imaginary number of infant deaths would be much lower.[61]

What is perhaps more interesting is that the chances of a person being hit by lightning are 1 in 13,000, of being killed in a car accident are 1 in 9,100, of drowning are 1 in 4,400, and the chances of developing a peanut allergy are 1 in 50. All of these have a much, much higher chance of causing infant deaths than breastsleeping, or even sharing a bed without breastfeeding. To better understand the odds of a death, the wider perspective is always useful. It is sometimes very surprising what risks we give attention to, and what risks we tend to ignore or perceive in vastly different ways.

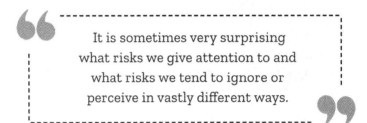

> It is sometimes very surprising what risks we give attention to and what risks we tend to ignore or perceive in vastly different ways.

Here is what we know. Mothers have coslept with their babies throughout human history, and it has proven evolutionarily beneficial for them to do so. Most nations with SIDS rates much lower than the United States regularly practice bedsharing on firm surfaces, with low rates of adult smoking, and high rates of breastfeeding. In other words, they are safely breastsleeping. Cosleeping is a tradition in at least 70% of all documented cultures, and it is universal across modern hunter-gatherer cultures. Most world cultures consider forcing babies to sleep apart from their mothers to be an act of cruelty or infant abuse.[62]

More and more U.S. families are making the decision to cosleep. More than half (61.4%) report cosleeping in some form, and more than one third do so "rarely or sometimes."[63] Since 1993, bedsharing in the U.S. has grown from about 6% of parents to 24% in 2015. As cosleeping rates rise, health care providers must be ready to entertain two-way, supportive conversations with parents about the practice so they can be instructed on how to do it safely.

In New Zealand, recommendations are tailored to each family and their specific circumstances, and they've experienced a 30% reduction in mortality since 2010.[64] They are not simply forbidding parents from cosleeping—they've found that many disregard that advice—but, rather, they're teaching parents how to do it safely. The United Kingdom has likewise been following a similar approach and has also seen a large drop in SIDS over the past few decades.

According to Dr. Blair, "We [in the U.K.] acknowledge that bedsharing happens both intentionally and unintentionally, and try to be non-judgmental; we don't strictly advise against it. We can discuss it openly with parents and advise them when it is really not a good idea. This approach was reviewed by our National Institute for Health & Care Excellence (NICE) in England in 2014 and the recommendation was to continue with our approach providing bidirectional, respectful conversations with parents."[50]

Parents are responsible for the care of a child, and their situations and goals must be respected. Educating parents, who can then make informed decisions, should be the role of all who advise and counsel families.

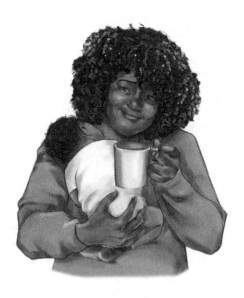

## CHAPTER 5

# "Never Cosleep!"

## Bedsharing and the American Academy of Pediatrics

The American Academy of Pediatrics (AAP) was founded in 1931 by 35 pediatricians, with the purpose of advocating for "optimal physical, mental, and social health and well-being for all infants, children, adolescents, and young adults."[65] Initially, the AAP did not fully recommend breastfeeding; the board only began to "strongly recommend" it in 1978, when the Committee on Nutrition issued a statement on breastfeeding in conjunction with the Nutrition Committee of the Canadian Pediatric Society. Since then, the AAP has progressively advocated for breastfeeding, skin-to-skin contact, and roomsharing, but has decided to rigidly advise against any and all bedsharing.

In 1994, the AAP launched the Back to Sleep® campaign with support and funding from the National Institute of Child Health and Human Development (NICHD), which advocated for the supine sleep position (positioned on back) for infants, rather than the prone position (positioned on stomach). This campaign was inspired by epidemiological studies conducted in New Zealand, led by Dr. Ed Mitchell, and in Great Britain, led by Dr. Fleming, with Dr. Blair as the statistician. It is credited for a decrease in the rate of SIDS deaths by over 50% by 2010, as well as a decrease in infants sleeping in prone position from 83% to 27%. When their policies come from a responsible, unbiased place, the AAP has tremendous potential to help families stay safe and healthy.

In addition to their influence in the media, the AAP advocates for their policies on the local, state, and federal level, making them a leading voice in shaping pediatric care at every stage. Their members lobby congress, monitor legislation, and build coalitions to promote their message. The AAP spent over $700,000 in 2017 lobbying Congress for various causes, such as child nutrition and increased aid for the water crisis in Flint, Michigan.

With encouragement from certain SIDS organizations, the AAP has unfortunately led the anti-bedsharing crusade.[66] When you hear that the American Academy of Pediatrics recommends against bedsharing, you might picture hundreds of learned SIDS research physicians all sharing ideas, opinions, and interpretations of data, but this is not the case. The Infant Sleep Position and SIDS Subcommittee, which I briefly talked about before, is comprised of 10–12 trained medical doctors and various external consultants when needed. To my knowledge, there is not any discipline diversity on the subcommittee, nor any individuals trained in psychobiology or the developmental or evolutionary sciences.

Through the years, I have gotten to know three or four of the committee members and have maintained a respectful, yet distant, relationship with them. At one time, before my scientific research took a different path from the committee, I was regularly asked to present plenary lectures at international SIDS conferences and was quite involved and thought to be a valuable resource in the world of SIDS prevention research. But, starting around 2005, it became clear that the subcommittee members were insistent and uncompromising in their belief that bedsharing is by default an unsafe sleep environment and is not to be supported. They were no longer interested in my research, or in the perspectives of anyone else who opposed their viewpoint.

The formulation of public health recommendations concerning complex, multi-faceted subjects like this, especially those with implications for civil liberties, ought not to consist of small insular groups all trained in the same ways. The AAP should have been holding its doors open for participation by the diverse constituencies affected by their decisions, including all scientists whose research perspectives and disciplines are relevant.

> The AAP should have been holding its doors open for participation by the diverse constituencies affected by their decisions.

Despite the massive holes in the information used to build their argument, the AAP's anti-bedsharing message holds a certain level of gravity. They have significant influence in shaping both cultural and medical attitudes, as well as civil and legal processes. For example, while I am not aware of the AAP encouraging U.S. Child Protective Services to threaten families who bedshare with taking away their infant, or to prosecute parents who lose an infant while bedsharing, I have also not seen evidence of the AAP or similar organizations releasing statements defending the rights of those families. These organizations have a responsibility to help protect good parents from threats by Child Protective Services, or from spouses or anyone else attempting to use the charge of "cosleeping" or "bedsharing" to take away custody of their infant or child.

Throughout my career, I have successfully submitted judicial-legal statements or testified under oath on behalf of far too many breastsleeping mothers, mothers sleeping with toddlers or older children, and parents who lost a child while bedsharing. I have been heartened by the fact that in not one of these instances did a mother lose custody after I was able to submit evidence supporting the fact that she was not harming her baby or child. Likewise, I was asked to testify in several trials dealing with alleged suffocations. Most recently, I testified for a father whose baby died while sleeping with him on a couch. The charge was "taking an infant to bed," leading to the infant's death. While I don't condone cosleeping on a couch, the specific charge the father was facing was clearly inappropriate. Upon reading all my materials, the prosecutor dismissed the charges in the middle of the trial.

My point is that it would be helpful, especially here in the U.S.—where parents can easily be mistreated by police, the courts, and Child Protective Services—for the AAP to make a clear and strong statement that it is not unlawful to bedshare, and that bedsharing parents following safety guidelines are not irresponsible.

This also entails recommending to hospitals that they should not pressure parents to avoid bedsharing, but rather should get involved in disseminating safety information about bedsharing in an open, objective, non-threatening way. Most importantly, hospitals should not be banning lactation counselors from sharing lifesaving information. They are on the front lines and have the most contact with new mothers and families. Policies that keep them from discussing bedsharing at all potentially lead to more, not fewer, sleep-related deaths, and put thousands of lactation counselors and nurses in conflict with their own ethical, moral, and professional values. Their jobs should not be in jeopardy for doing the very thing they are trained for: keeping mothers and babies safe by promoting breastfeeding and safe infant sleep.

Physicians' advice to parents also closely follows the AAP's recommendations, and studies show that mothers trust the advice of their physicians more than that of nurses, family, or friends. However, despite the negative marketing, mothers are still choosing to bedshare at a growing rate. So why is this?

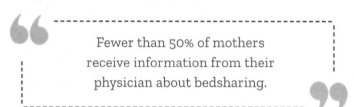

> Fewer than 50% of mothers receive information from their physician about bedsharing.

The disconnect is a result of the AAP's infant sleep guidelines being one-size-fits-all in nature, and mothers recognizing that shortcoming in the information they are given. A longitudinal study conducted over 23 years found that fewer than 50% of mothers receive information from their physician about bedsharing, and, of the mothers who do get information, 73% report receiving negative advice.[67] As a consequence, parents are rarely properly informed on safe bedsharing practices.

In spite of their efforts to promote safe sleep practices, the AAP's success in reducing SIDS and SUID will remain plateaued so long as they dismiss the significant role that bedsharing plays in supporting breastfeeding and regulating infant physiology and behavior, as will be discussed in Part 3.

While the AAP advocates for mothers to breastfeed their infants for at least one full year, their recommendations against bedsharing actually undermine any mother's ability to accomplish this goal. Breastsleeping is the very strategy by which many mothers, according to their own reports, can achieve their goal of extended breastfeeding. In addition, AAP recommendations ignore factors like individual infant sleep personalities, infant temperaments, and the underlying biology controlling infant and parent emotions, explained by an evolutionary perspective.

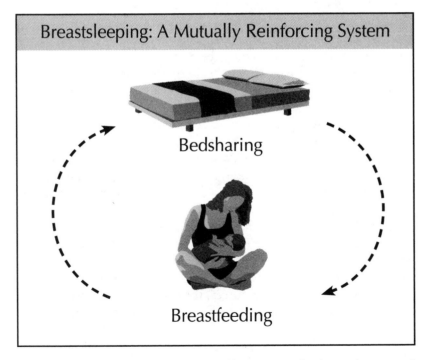

## Breastsleeping: A Mutually Reinforcing System

Bedsharing

Breastfeeding

*Fig. 2.7 Bedsharing and breastfeeding strongly support each other in the ease and continuation of both practices. Bedsharing makes it easier and more practical to breastfeed regularly, and breastfeeding makes it safer and more practical to bedshare.*

In Brigitte Jordan's classic book, *Birth in Four Cultures,* she described some of the problems and controversies relevant to what she called "medical authoritative knowledge." Jordan addressed these issues in the context of the increasing "medicalization of birthing" as it occurs in Western industrialized societies. The rise of medical authoritative knowledge and its inherent limitations assert the same set of constraints for SIDS scientists, including myself and the colleagues I have mentioned thus far, specializing in a variety of research disciplines.

Jordan describes authoritative medical knowledge as legitimizing one way of understanding research while devaluing or dismissing all other ways of understanding. She says, "Those who reject authoritative knowledge systems tend to be seen as backward, ignorant, or naïve troublemakers....The power of authoritative medicine is not that it is correct, but that it counts." One outcome of Western medical authoritative knowledge is that the AAP has successfully controlled the discourse on infant care.

The AAP perspective is that bedsharing is always dangerous, so they dismiss the validity of maternal instincts and agency and the legitimate choices made by millions of mothers here in the U.S. and abroad. Parents' experiences and emotions offer important insight into the difficulties and inconsistencies encountered while navigating the question and practice of where their baby will sleep, but their voices are not given enough weight in the conversation. The same can be said for a variety of highly relevant scientific findings offered by many disciplines, especially those which offer powerful enriching perspectives and explanations for what is missing in the present recommendations, and how and why they need to change.

In making the eradication of any and all bedsharing their primary goal, the AAP reviewed lines of evidence with a selective bias that reflects Western social values of individualism and faith in technology over maternal bodies. With institutional outreach and sufficient monetary resources, they are able to undermine any alternatives to medical authoritative knowledge, replacing it solely with their own supposedly evidence-based knowledge, which, as it turns out, falls significantly short of the standards of Evidence-Based Medicine.

>

# How Current Recommendations
# Bypass Evidence-Based Medicine

*"Evidence-Based Medicine is not 'cookbook' medicine.... Any external guideline must be integrated with individual clinical expertise in deciding whether and how it matches the patient's clinical state, predicament, and preferences."*

—DR. DAVID L. SACKETT[68]

As journalist H.L. Mencken once said, "There is always a well-known solution to every human problem—neat, plausible, and wrong."[69] If there were ever a line that best described what has happened in the bedsharing debate, this is it.

I have already talked about how current thinking on cosleeping reflects only a small segment of evidence available from many different fields of study. Here, I will explain why I have been very critical of the process by which organizations like the AAP and the National Institute of Child Health and Human Development (NICHD) have formulated their safe sleep recommendations.

First and foremost, as we touched upon in Chapter 4, they have violated the basic principles of Evidence-Based Medicine, starting with their failure to ask what the patients want, think, and need. Dr. David Sackett, known as the father of EBM, defined the practice as the integration of "thoughtful identification and compassionate use of individual patients' predicaments, rights, and preferences in making clinical decisions about their care," with the "best available external clinical evidence."[68]

According to Dr. Sackett himself, the EBM approach is anything but top-down medicine. In fact, it is bottom-up, as it begins with how patients think and how they express or value certain ideas about their health and their children's health. According to Dr. Sackett and colleagues, the patient's perspective and interpretations of scientific findings or debates are primary. The U.S. Institute of Medicine's Committee on Quality of Health Care in America also emphasized in their 2001 publication that, for effective evidence-based practice, patient values "must be integrated into clinical decisions."[70]

EBM requires individual clinical judgments to be determined

by health professionals who work directly with families.

Dr. Sackett says, "It is this expert that decides whether the external evidence applies to the individual patient at all, and, if so, how it should be integrated into a clinical decision."[68] Individual healthcare providers should be the ones to determine, on a case-by-case basis, through conversations with their patients, to what degree standard recommendations are appropriate.

In the making of broad public health recommendations, careful attention must be given to circumstances that change the appropriateness of a practice, procedure, or treatment. Dr. Sackett and colleagues make it clear that "external clinical evidence can inform, but can never replace, individual clinical expertise," meaning that general public health recommendations should not be presented as the singular, hard-lined rule. This is important for maximizing adherence to the recommendation. Parents are more likely to follow guidelines if they can do it in a way that works for their family.

> General public health recommendations should not be presented as the singular, hard-lined rule.

Furthermore, according to the principles of EBM, epidemiological findings should not be immediately turned into sweeping public health messages. First, hypotheses about how to explain patterns in the data must be tested. This is especially true when the studies reveal inconsistency in the data, which is one way of saying that the same behavior can have vastly different outcomes depending on the presence or absence of certain co-factors.

Knowing that the safety of bedsharing depends entirely on such co-factors, extra care should have been taken to thoroughly test any relevant hypotheses before recommendations were made. This was not the case. The AAP and NICHD continue to ignore the fact that there are many modifiable factors that contribute to the safety of bedsharing, instead choosing to condemn the practice in all its forms, as if they all share the same level of risk.

Searching for consensus and inviting all relevant scientists into the conversation is also a central part of Evidence-Based

Medicine. As we know, the AAP and NICHD have not sought to do this, ignoring disagreements from scientists with legitimate research in related, but non-medical fields. My own 30 years of anthropological and physiological research dedicated to this subject has been repeatedly dismissed. Lactation counselors and consultants have also been excluded from playing any significant, continuing role in the formulation of recommendations. They are the primary touchpoints for millions of breastfeeding mothers worldwide, with unique and remarkable insights into the practical challenges families face; as such, their perspective should be given more weight.

Let's put it this way. Making appropriate recommendations on sleeping arrangements based on the practice of EBM would mean two things. First of all, all practitioners would be expected to understand the unique circumstances each family faces, and to consider the needs and wants of parents before making specific recommendations to them. Second, the recommendations of the AAP and NICHD would be based on the most up-to-date and comprehensive research available, not on epidemiological studies alone or on research that fails to identify all of the hazardous co-factors relevant to understanding bedsharing risk.

Finally, AAP representatives have been claiming for years that they cannot support bedsharing because they simply do not know how to make it safe. Yet, to my knowledge, the AAP and the NICHD have never requested funding or allotted research money to studies to address this question. My guess is that they have to first appreciate and value a behavior before investing time and money into researching it. But parents *do* value breastsleeping, and the practice is not going away any time soon. We know what the important questions are, and I believe it is the responsibility of influential health institutions to lead the way in answering them with current, comprehensive studies, rather than continuing to say *we just don't know.*

Considering their disregard for the tried and true principles of EBM, it is not a surprise that, for 20 years, these institutions have failed to convince breastsleeping mothers, and millions of other families, that bedsharing somehow undermines their child's health.

>

# What Public Health Officials and Civil Authorities Might Tell You

*"Don't sleep with your baby or put the baby down in an adult bed. The only safe place for a baby to sleep is in a crib that meets current safety standards and has a firm, tight-fitting mattress."*

—ANN BROWN, FORMER CPSC CHAIRMAN[71]

In 1999, the U.S. Consumer Product Safety Commission Chairman, Ann Brown, called a multi-media news conference featuring authors of a newly published study of babies who died from apparent accidental suffocation.[72] This study counted deaths that occurred in a variety of sleeping arrangements, including alone in an adult bed, alongside other persons, alone in a crib, or sleeping beside adults in chairs, recliners, or waterbeds. The locations and circumstances of the deaths were not discussed during the news conference. While the majority of deaths in the study by far occurred when infants slept alone, the intention of the conference was not to point out the reality of how dangerous it is for babies to sleep outside the supervision of a caregiver. The focus was exclusively on babies dying in adult beds, and the goal was to warn parents against any and all bedsharing. The programming included a video of a parent likened to a wooden rolling pin, inert and unmoving, laying passively over an infant while the narrator sternly warned something along the lines of, *it only takes ten seconds to suffocate your baby.*

The study was missing data and did not clearly define suffocation deaths. It also lacked the information needed to understand the relative risk of each sleep location included in the study, both in comparison to each other and to the total number of babies whose parents practiced each sleeping arrangement. Nevertheless, the authors concluded that bedsharing was far more dangerous than solitary sleeping for infants. At the time, this conclusion was widely criticized, as no adequate data was put forward to be able to draw such a conclusion.

Since 1999, when Ann Brown called her news conference, the anti-bedsharing messaging has become increasingly clearer and more threatening: Sleeping with your baby is dangerous, and should absolutely not be allowed under any circumstances.

In May 2002, the U.S. Consumer Product Safety Commission published a news release reinforcing the anti-cosleeping message. The Juvenile Products Manufacturers Association (in other words, the crib industry) offered their conference as a forum for CPSC to make their announcement, and offered to help finance continuing promotion of the idea to doctors and stores.[73] The crib industry went further by providing "Safe Sleep" brochures to major toy stores and other venues, creating a video clip for wide media distribution, and granting continued "education" on the topic to physicians.[66]

"Sharing an adult bed with an infant is not cool, nor is it an indicator of educated parenting,"[74] said Marian Sokol, President of the SIDS Alliance, following the 2005 death of a bedsharing infant whose teen mother had consumed 18 cans of beer before getting into bed.

In 2008, the director of the L.A. County Inter-Agency Council on Child Abuse and Neglect, Deanne Tilton Durfee, stated, "We know the value of holding your child, cuddling your child, loving your child. But if you take the baby to bed with you and fall asleep, you are committing a potentially lethal act."[75]

Spokespersons would add something like: *No responsible parent who wants the best for their baby would ever sleep in a bed with them.* However, with millions of mothers from many Western countries sleeping on the same surface with their babies, either more mothers are "irresponsible" than would be expected, or responsible mothers simply reject claims that bedsharing cannot be done safely.

But still, this singular, unqualified, and unyielding message continues to be applied to millions of parents who are expected to follow the rules or face societal consequences—from the "bad parent" label to more tangible, frightening legal consequences.

Of course, the goal is noble: to eliminate sleep-related infant deaths. But to attempt to take a fundamental civil liberty and a species-defining attribute away from parents is not the way to do this. Who gave any committee permission to attempt to eradicate something so important to human beings? Where a baby sleeps is not a medical issue at its core, but a relational one. For many parents, it reflects how they want to protect, communicate, and express their love for their infants.

Like most widespread marketing campaigns, the methods used to achieve this goal are extreme and generic, and certainly not tailored to meet the needs of individual families. Sokol's statement that mothers are "uneducated" if they bedshare is absolutely inappropriate. And, for the record, I have never met a bedsharing mother that bedshares to be "cool," as Sokol suggests. Tilton Durfee's comment that parents who bring their baby to bed are committing a "lethal" act is also wholly inappropriate in its threatening implications.

> Where a baby sleeps is not a medical issue at its core, but a relational one.

Certainly, these remarks show no regard for the parents' inherent right to interpret studies and evidence for themselves, as well as their right to make an educated and thoughtful decision about bedsharing.[37] At best, these well-intended public expressions are simply wrong, and patently condescending to boot. They are themselves—to use Sokol's description—"uneducated" responses, both because they fail to account for other lines of evidence that refute them and because they fail to resonate with families' experiences worldwide.

In 2011, the city of Milwaukee began an anti-cosleeping campaign using photos of babies tucked into adult beds alongside wicked-looking knives (see Appendix V). Text above the images declares, "Your baby sleeping with you can be just as dangerous."[76] Milwaukee health officials were telling parents that sleeping in the same bed as their baby was as dangerous as allowing them to sleep beside a meat cleaver. Christie Haskell, writing for *The Stir*, wrote, "Before anyone insists this campaign is brilliant,…consider if it were a bottle of formula labeled as poison. This isn't any different."[77]

That same year, less than two months after the initial launch of the campaign, two more Milwaukee infants died in sleep-related accidents. The press was quick to label these tragedies as the same kind of inevitable "cosleeping deaths" the campaign was trying—and apparently failing—to prevent. The truth is, both infants had been sleeping with multiple other children, in chaotic, unsafe environments. They were not sleeping with the protection of a sober, breastfeeding mother, in a deliberate bedsharing environment, free from other hazards. Both arrangements may be considered cosleeping, or bedsharing, but the unsafe nature of one sleeping arrangement does not mean the other, very different arrangement must also be unsafe.

While the cause of death for these infants does not make the situation any less horrific, it does say something about the misrepresentation of facts in these types of campaigns, and the common oversimplification of an extremely complex issue. According to an essay about this incident by Dr. Kathleen Kendall-Tackett, "The sad take-away we can learn from these cases is that 'simple messages' may be headline-grabbing. But in the end, they lack credibility, and do not communicate what parents need to know to keep their infants safe while sleeping."[78]

Today, safe sleep campaigns across the country continue to use images and slogans intended to frighten new parents into compliance. No doubt you have seen some of them (if not, see Appendix V). This includes posters showing the headboard of an adult bed grimly edited to look like a tombstone, etched with the words: "For too many babies last year, this was their final resting place." If the shock value of these campaigns isn't enough, the "ABC" acronym developed by small-scale Safe to Sleep campaigns is hammered into the minds of new parents: "Alone, Back, Crib." Two of the three guidelines are specifically targeted to stop cosleeping practices. With such a clear, one-sided message, it would seem that cosleeping deaths should be on the decline, yet, unfortunately, they are not.

The AAP's 1994 Back to Sleep® campaign was hugely successful, leading to a significant decline in SUID rates. So, when the AAP next turned to bedsharing and labeled the practice as "hazardous," other health authorities were quick to jump on board. Major organizations in the U.S., including the Federal SIDS/SUID Work Group, Centers for Disease Control and Prevention (CDC), the Eunice Kennedy Shriver National Institute of Child Health and Human Development (NICHD), the American SIDS Institute, the Children's Safety Network (CSN), and the National Action Partnership to Promote Safe Sleep (NAPPSS) followed the AAP's lead, unanimously condemning bedsharing in the hopes of reducing sleep-related deaths. However, this time, the campaigns seemed to have the opposite effect of what these groups intended.

Accidental suffocation deaths, most often credited to cosleeping or, more specifically, bedsharing, started to increase. The death rate peaked in 2015, with 23.1 deaths per 100,000 infants,[79] even though bedsharing had unofficially been included as a safety hazard in the AAP discussions since 2000. Theoretically, after 15 years of anti-bedsharing campaigns, the death rate should have decreased. Instead, it was increasing. Clearly, something was not adding up.

Anti-bedsharing messaging has failed to stop the practice of bedsharing in any of its forms, both safe and unsafe, and has also failed to reduce infant deaths despite being fiercely reinforced by all major infant health agencies and authorities. Indeed, recent studies show that threats and sweeping, negative messaging are giving rise to new hazards.

---

## Why the Message Doesn't Work

Picture an exhausted mother. It's 2 AM and she is waking up—yet again—to the cries of her hungry baby. She throws back the sheets and clambers out of bed to make her way to the crib. She picks up the baby to breastfeed, but is so tired she can barely stay standing.

Now this mother has two options. She can either lie down in bed to breastfeed, or sit on a couch or a chair. Even in her sleep-deprived fog, she remembers the message: *Do not bedshare. Bedsharing is dangerous.* Think, again, of Deanne Tilton Durfee's condemnation of parents who "take the baby to bed."

Instead of taking the baby back to bed with her, the mother decides to sit for just a moment on the couch. She tells herself she will put the baby back in the crib as soon as she is finished feeding, and then she will go to bed. Just a few minutes later, she leans back into the couch and her eyelids begin to drift shut....

It is well known and clearly proven that falling asleep on a couch or recliner with a baby is significantly more likely to have fatal consequences than sleeping in a bed. Even the AAP agrees that couches are a more dangerous sleep surface than beds. Their recommendations state that parents should lie in bed to breastfeed during the night, rather than sit on the couch where the risk is much greater if they happen to fall asleep.

> The more authorities push against bedsharing, the more parents are afraid of it, and the more likely they are to fall asleep in dangerous cosleeping arrangements.

However, it seems to be a logical assumption that it is more likely for a mother to fall asleep while breastfeeding in bed, as opposed to sitting up on the couch. Regardless of whether that assumption is true, the message from authorities is so strongly opposed to sleeping in bed with a baby that many parents will think nighttime feedings are safer on the couch or a recliner.

Infant deaths caused by falling asleep on a couch, chair, or recliner are grouped under the umbrella term of "cosleeping deaths," or sometimes "bedsharing deaths," when clearly they are not. Health authorities then use these numbers as "evidence" pointing to the dangers of bedsharing, without making the necessary distinctions as to where and how the deaths took place, instead lumping them into the same generic bin. Ironically, the more authorities push against bedsharing, the more parents are afraid of it, and the more likely they are to fall asleep in dangerous cosleeping arrangements. A 20-year population-based study by Dr. Peter Blair and colleagues observed that, as total SIDS cases decreased, there was a notable increase in the number of deaths caused by sleeping with an infant on the sofa.[80]

Even if a mother follows recommendations to avoid the couch and to lie in bed for nighttime feedings, what is she supposed to do in the event that she falls asleep there? If she looks for advice from any public health authority, she will find that the only way to keep her baby safe is to not fall asleep.

Imagine this suggestion: In their "Safe Sleep" instructions, the Illinois Department of Children and Family Services actually states, "If you breastfeed in bed, soothe your baby back to sleep while standing, and return her to the crib when she is asleep."[81]

Standing up in a hallway or bedroom to soothe your baby back to sleep? If they really believe this will happen, they need a quick course in human behavioral biology. I think it goes without saying that this is not a plausible rule for parents to follow.

In a 2010 study of nighttime sleep locations, 70% of mothers who fed their babies in bed said they were likely to fall asleep there.[37] Lactation consultant and author Linda J. Smith says it best when she states, "Sleep happens, and exhaustion overrules common sense...."[82] Professional advice suggesting to stand or keep yourself awake in bed fails to understand or respect the sometimes overwhelming power of biology. Mothers are supposed to fall asleep while next to their infants. And, hence, they do.

Dr. Blair says: "I can see why a simple message not to bedshare might be a tempting strategy. Reducing the primary risk factors that affect bedsharing safety, which are generally smoking and alcohol consumption, is no easy task. If there is little cultural value placed on the practice, or a lack of other perceived advantages, it might be the path of least resistance."[50] That said, according to mothers themselves and judging from the millions of mothers now choosing to breastsleep, a seismic cultural shift has taken place.

Despite the fear tactics and negative messaging, many parents, both breastfeeding and non-breastfeeding, choose to intentionally bedshare with their babies. Looking back at the sleep location study from 2010,[37] bedsharing rates over an infant's first year were as high as 62%, with mothers who were exclusively breastfeeding being the most likely to bedshare consistently. About 69% of the bedsharing mothers involved in the survey indicated that it was the only sleeping arrangement that worked for their family.

A randomized controlled trial published by the AAP in 2016 looked at enhanced messaging targeted to black American mothers to deter them from bedsharing. Even in trial conditions, the bedsharing rates actually went slightly up rather than significantly down.[83] Similarly, a different study conducted among at-risk American mothers found that, even with full knowledge of the AAP's definition of safe sleep, 100% of these mothers rejected or failed to adhere to the AAP recommendations.[84]

Increasingly, research is also revealing a ubiquitous response to the question of *why do you bedshare?* What most mothers say is:

*to get more sleep.* Even in light of the increased effort required of bedsharing caregivers, especially breastfeeding ones, mothers still turn to bedsharing to reduce their exhaustion, to better manage their milk supply, and to improve the restfulness of their babies, as well as to more strongly attach with them.[16, 36] Dr. Blair states, "It is clear that many American and European mothers do value bedsharing, not only for practical reasons like getting more sleep and managing their milk supply, but also for emotional ones."[50]

A caseworker for New York's Office of Children and Family Services (OCFS)—a self-described "foot soldier" for the enforcement of state-endorsed safe infant sleep policies—offered comments for a story that my colleague, Dr. Lee Gettler, and I wrote for *Mothering Magazine* in 2010.[85] The employee, going by the name P. Angie, had some regrets about his role in the state's anti-bedsharing campaign.

The campaign, called "Babies Sleep Safest Alone" at the time (the OCFS now uses the popular "ABCs of Safe Sleep" messaging), claimed that any and all bedsharing is extremely dangerous. Angie argued, "This blanket approach is out of step with a belief commonly held in social services that all families are unique, presenting different situations and strengths."

Even with an insider's perspective, it was clear that there are a variety of issues endemic to anti-bedsharing recommendations. Education is a more effective strategy than "asking mom, dad, and baby to stop bedsharing, buy a crib, and change their entire nighttime routine," which Angie suggests "is highly intrusive, and is a request more likely to be ignored or only appear to be followed—for instance, by buying a crib and not using it." Parents can be taught relatively simple but important actions concerning bedsharing safety that can make a real difference. The caseworker pointed out, "Changes that are the least disruptive preserve the integrity of a family and are more likely to be followed."

Perhaps this is why negative comments, warnings, and messages have been unsuccessful. They collectively fail because those constructing the messages do not appreciate why mothers bedshare, or the powerful emotional and biological mechanisms that make sleeping with one's baby (especially if breastfeeding) legitimate, sometimes necessary, and often desirable.

I am inclined to believe that parents who intentionally choose to bedshare do so because it is the best arrangement for their family, and no clinician will ever be able to convince them otherwise.

In sum, I think it's reasonable to say that the current Safe to Sleep campaign message is missing its mark. It is the perfect time, then, for the increasingly popular parental safety practice of cosleeping to become an integral part of a more empathetic and comprehensive set of evidence-based recommendations. This could transition the "bedsharing debate" into a bidirectional discourse that can take place between all interested scientists and, more importantly, between health professionals and the families they serve.[1]

# Part 3

Everything You Need to Know
About Cosleeping

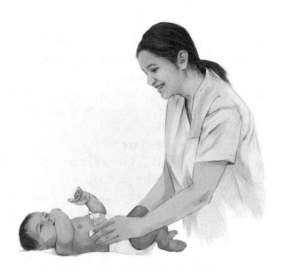

## CHAPTER 6

# The Science Behind Cosleeping

## What Makes Breastsleeping Safe?

My support of cosleeping, or, more specifically, breastsleeping, as the safest and most natural way for a human baby to sleep stems from my research on how and why it occurs, what it means to mothers, how it functions biologically, and its evolutionary history.[11, 16, 33] Like human taste buds, which reward us for eating what's overwhelmingly critical for survival (i.e. fat, salt, and sugar), a consideration of human infant and parent biology and psychology reveals the existence of powerful physiological and social factors that motivate and reward us for cosleeping. This explains why parents feel the need to touch and sleep close to their babies.[31, 86, 87]

Infants usually have something to say about where they sleep, too—and for some reason they remain unimpressed with declarations as to how dangerous sleeping next to mother can be, or how important it is that they learn to be independent. Mother's body is the only environment for which the infant is truly adapted, and for which even modern Western technology has yet to produce a substitute. Prominent physician and neuroscientist Dr. Nils Bergman describes the mother's body as the human infant's "habitat;"[88] nothing a baby can or cannot do makes sense except in light of this.

Despite dramatic cultural and technological changes in the industrialized West, we know that human infants are still born the most neurologically immature primate, with only 25% of their adult brain volume.[24] This brain immaturity relates to the underdevelopment of their immune, respiratory, cognitive, and digestive systems, their chewing abilities, and their control over movement or vocalizations. At birth, our species-wide reflexes dominate over our ability to make judgments and decisions. In those first few months of life, humans are the closest we will get to the direct, universal expression of our genetic instincts, because, of course, infants are not aware of any particular culture. We see the same exact bodily responses during breastsleeping across the world, and a universal instinct for infants to elicit close contact from a caregiver.

> Breastsleeping is biologically driven.

Breastsleeping is biologically driven, both by an infant's need for nutrition in the form of breastmilk and by its inherent need for physical contact. Staying close to the mother or other caregiver helps engage an infant's senses, which provides critical regulatory effects that protect the infant and compensate for extreme vulnerability.[28, 32, 33, 35, 47]

Neurologically-based infant responses to maternal warmth, smells (like mother's milk), movements, and touch reduce infant crying while positively regulating breathing, body temperature, absorption of calories, stress hormone levels, immune status, and oxygenation. In short, it seems to make babies happy. So, unless practiced dangerously (see Chapter 8), sleeping next to mother either on the same or a different surface is overwhelmingly good for babies and is what their bodies were designed to experience. But what is it that makes cosleeping not only beneficial, but safe?

Based on their immaturity and need for closeness from a caregiver, human infants have developed strategies to protect themselves. As British psychologist John Bowlby argued years ago in his classic formulation of the concept of maternal-infant attachment, the social bond that develops between a mother and her infant is the result of evolved infant reflexes and attributes reducing the chances of maternal abandonment. Among these are behaviors designed to elicit the care they need to survive—evoking what animal behavior researchers call the "cute response" by way of traits which attract us to infants and make us want to respond to and protect them. These behaviors include infants moving in excitement when seeing someone familiar, and looking or smiling at them, and eventually following, grasping at, and moving toward caregivers.[89] Anthropologist Sarah Blaffer Hrdy proposes that babies developed physical features such as soft rounded cheeks, baby fat, relatively big, rounded eyes, sweet vocalizations, and other "cute" characteristics so mothers will invest in, care for, and attach to them.[23]

Infants, also have more practical survival adaptations. Since human infants are unable to regulate their body temperature by shivering, they have had to evolve ways to protect themselves from the cold. The instinct to use mother's body to keep warm is one of those ways, but human infants are also born with insulation in the form of about 9–15% body fat, which is higher than any other primate. Moreover, energy-producing brown fat tissue is distributed on the human newborn's neck, back, and shoulders that may have evolved to calorically sustain the baby between the time he or she is born and when mother's breastmilk first comes in.

Infants have also developed the ability to react to and alert their caregivers of dangerous situations. Contrary to what you might infer from anti-bedsharing messages, babies do not lie still and keep quiet when something is wrong or hurting them. An experiment in the '70s recorded how healthy newborns reacted to having their airways obstructed. While the procedure is ethically problematic, it did clearly indicate that even day-old newborns are not just protoplasmic blobs lying there waiting to be suffocated by someone.

According to the researchers, "Most infants respond by opening their mouths...and by pushing out with the tongue or yawning. When this proves ineffective in getting rid of the stimulus, more vigorous movements begin, involving head rocking from side to side, head retractions, back arching in avoidance, and, lastly, head batting of (or at) the stimulus. Frequent mouth and head responses will occur simultaneously." The researchers concluded that it was quite easy for infants to rid themselves of dangerous blockages "because of the vigor of defensive responses newborn infants make."[90]

This description is certainly dramatic, but, despite being uncomfortable to read, it accurately demonstrates that a normal newborn has every capacity to at least let a sober breastsleeping or cosleeping companion know when something is very wrong.

Legendary SIDS researcher Dr. Marie Valdes-Dapena, who studied tens of thousands of infants who died from SIDS, stated, "A normal sleeping adult will be aroused by the struggles of an over-lain infant before suffocation occurs unless, of course, the adult is inebriated or under the influence of drugs."[91] She suggests that mothers are designed to respond to such dramatic infantile reactions, or even less dramatic signals. Parents are more than biologically prepared to respond appropriately and immediately to any signals of distress, as long as they are sober and invested. I find it offensive when medical professionals try to say that a mother—no matter who she is or what her circumstances are—poses an inherent risk to her baby by merely lying on the same surface for sleep.

I acknowledge that the majority of new mothers in the world are, at the very least, very, very tired. However, this does not translate to mothers being automatically unable to detect the presence of their baby next to them in bed, or unable to avoid an overlaying accident.

Let's go back a step or two. Our species' greatest protection, which co-evolved with sleep itself, is being able to awaken quickly. Humans remain highly attuned, sensitive, and responsive to the nighttime environment while asleep. We have the evolved ability to evacuate a sleep site if necessary; to respond to unexpected noises, smells, and movements; and to confront any number of attacks by micro and macro predators alike. In the case of our early ancestors, these included poisonous spiders, beetles, snakes, eagles, hyenas, leopards, jackals, or saber-tooth cats, against which our only real defense was anticipation, concealment, and our social collective actions to ward them off.

In earlier evolutionary times, before 1–1.5 million years ago and before the discovery and control of fire, our upright walking human ancestors likely did not sleep on the ground. Instead, they would have nested themselves and their babies up in trees at night to be less vulnerable to nocturnal predators. Like our present-day infants, these early ancestral infants would have been born relatively immature, without muscles for clinging to their mother's chests. This meant that mothers needed, more than ever, to hold tightly to their infants throughout the night to prevent them from falling out of trees or from unstable cliff dwellings. This made it critical, for both infant and adult survival, to develop a level of consciousness during sleep and a high degree of maternal, sleep-related monitoring abilities.[38, 47, 54]

Our behavioral and physiological studies of contemporary bedsharing mothers and infants documented this exact thing. Mothers are able to awaken quickly from sleep in response to what an infant is doing or not doing, and vice versa (infants awaken in relationship to what their mother is doing). We found that breastsleeping mothers and infants were highly sensitive to each other's awakenings. Of the total arousal pattern of both mothers and infants, we found in one study that approximately 40% of an infant's brief awakenings occurred plus or minus two seconds following their mother's arousal. Out of the total number of maternal arousals, over 60% of them occurred plus or minus two seconds following their infant's arousal, altogether reflecting a high degree of responsiveness during sleep even when mothers were in the deepest stage of sleep.[33, 87]

> Mothers are able to awaken quickly from sleep in response to what an infant is doing or not doing.

Not surprisingly, cosleeping also significantly increases the total number of nightly infant arousals. The baby gets a lot of practice in waking to the movements, awakenings, external sounds, and touches from his or her mother. This increase in arousals may help develop stronger and quicker awakening skills that can prove handy should the infant's oxygen supply decrease following a breathing pause. For breastsleeping pairs, the smell of mother's breastmilk nearby also contributes to the infant's tendency to remain in light sleep for a longer period of time.[8, 11, 87]

Compared to solitary-sleeping or formula-feeding babies, breastsleeping babies spend more time in Stage 1 and Stage 2 of sleep, rather than the deeper Stages 3 and 4. Light sleep is thought to be physiologically more appropriate for young infants. It is easier for babies to awaken from light stages of sleep than from deep stages of sleep, which again can be helpful when infants experience breathing pauses (apneas) or other dangers. Shorter durations of deep sleep can even help protect those infants born with arousal deficiencies, which are suspected to be involved in SIDS.[8, 11, 19, 46]

In addition to altering the sleep architecture of both mother and baby, cosleeping—especially in the form of breastsleeping—provides on-going "hidden regulatory mechanisms" that are not easily observed. According to research by Dr. Myron Hofer,

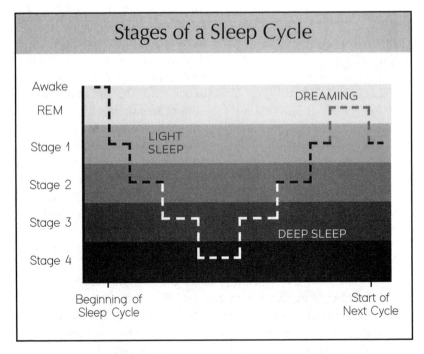

*Fig. 3.1 A depiction of a normal human sleep cycle. Infants who breastsleep spend more time in Stage 1 and Stage 2 of sleep, compared to solitary-sleeping infants. Babies in light stages of sleep are easier to arouse in case of apneas or arousal deficiencies.*

psychiatrist and expert on developmental psychobiology, these mechanisms exist specifically to compensate for the immature biological systems of newborn mammals, helping them successfully transition to life outside the womb.[92]

Take breathing, for example. Work by biobehavioral scientist Dr. Evelyn B. Thoman from the University of Connecticut showed that human infants are extremely sensitive to the chest movements and sounds of breathing companions. She and her colleague did a study on apnea-prone newborns placed next to artificially "breathing" mechanical teddy bears. The bears had pumps inserted into their chests, timed to rise and fall at the optimal breathing rate for each particular infant. The infants had, on average, 60% fewer stop-breathing episodes when they

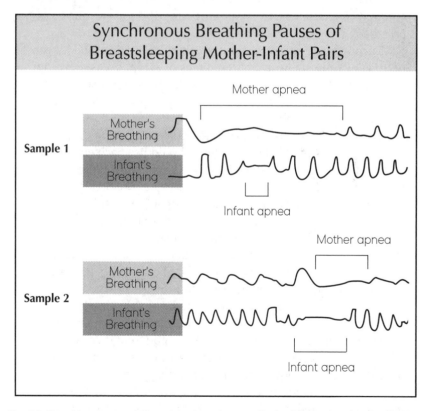

*Fig. 3.2 Breathing pauses (apneas) and awakenings for bedsharing mothers and infants tend to occur at the same time, or within 2 seconds of each other. This is can be seen in polygraphic tracings from a study I worked on with Dr. Sarah Mosko, published in 1990.*

were laid next to these breathing teddy bears.[93] Another study showed that other mammals, such as cats, also modify their sleep respiratory patterns based on the sounds they hear.[94]

Cosleeping infants might also experience steady breathing due to little puffs of carbon dioxide ($CO_2$) expelled by the mother's exhalation. When this $CO_2$ is inhaled by the closely positioned infant, it can potentially trigger enhanced responses of the nerve that drives the diaphragm, stimulating the lungs to release or exhale to get rid of the $CO_2$.

Hence, live, human breathing companions not only provide infants with rising and falling movement stimuli and audible breathing sounds (like the breathing teddy bears), but also provide these puffs of $CO_2$ that promote more stable breathing. Perhaps the exhaled breath caressing the infant's cheeks is another potential "hidden regulatory factor," nudging the baby to continue to breathe.[93, 95]

Through increased arousals, breathing regulation, and longer periods of time spent in lighter stages of sleep, breastsleeping naturally protects against SIDS. Ironically, these are also the same effects associated with pacifier use, though a pacifier doesn't have the added benefits of sensory stimuli.

Those AAP panelists opposed to bedsharing argue that, after breastfeeding is established, mothers should use pacifiers as one possible way to prevent SIDS. However, to my knowledge, it has never been confirmed whether falling asleep at the breast offers the same amount of protection as falling asleep while using a pacifier. It would be nice if everyone could have as much faith in what a mother's body can contribute to infant health as they do in the power of imitation nipples. I speculate that nursing at a real breast, rather than using a pacifier, should be all that is necessary to protect against SIDS, in addition to providing other kinds of sensory stimuli that are also important for healthy development.

I am sure it is already clear to you that one of the most important results of bedsharing is the promotion of breastfeeding. We know that breastfeeding provides a whole suite of health benefits for both mother and baby, including positive influences on brain growth and protection against any number of diseases, including SIDS and even forms of childhood cancers (see Chapter 7: Benefits of Cosleeping). But, along with these protective health benefits, there are also key differences in the way that breastfeeding mother-infant pairs sleep when compared to those who bottle-feed. Breastfeeding pairs develop conditioned safety habits and heightened mutual sensitivities that protect against the risk of overlaying.

I am more concerned about the safety of bedsharing for bottle-feeding mother-baby pairs because they do not display the same degree of conditioned mutual sensitivity that breastsleeping pairs do, and they do not show the same dramatic differences in overall sleep architecture, such as more light-stage sleep.[19] The behaviors and responses of breastsleeping mothers and infants tips the risk assessment toward acceptably safe, at least in the minds of those who study breastsleeping and are interested in documenting why bedsharing outcomes can vary so much.[16, 33, 47]

> I am more concerned about the safety of bedsharing for bottle-feeding pairs because they do not display the conditioned mutual sensitivity of breastsleeping pairs.

For example, breastfeeding mothers practically always place their babies in the safest sleep position—on their backs—without instruction. Sleeping supine is the only way a breastfeeding baby can get to and from the breast. Compared with bottle-feeding pairs, breastsleeping mothers tend to exhibit a universal side position with the baby at mid-chest level, under her triceps, with her legs curled up under the baby's feet. Their instinctual positioning turns the mother's body into a protective barrier, with inward-facing arms and legs preventing the mother from rolling toward the infant.

Breastsleeping mothers and babies also spend most of the night facing each other, a position that lends itself to social engagements and communication opportunities, which may enhance cognitive development. Due to increased sensitivity to the mother's body, combined with the scent of breastmilk, breastfed infants tend to stay in this safe position instead of moving away into potentially dangerous bed locations. Dr. Helen Ball may have been the first person to comment about the body positions of mother-baby pairs, and to call this breastsleeping position universal.

Directing the University of Durham Infancy and Sleep Centre in Great Britain, Dr. Ball specifically studied differences between bottle-feeding and breastfeeding dyads. According to her research,

| Characteristic Differences Among Breast and Formula-Fed Infants | | |
|---|---|---|
| **Average Orientation to Mother** | **Formula-Fed** | **Breastfed** |
| Mother facing infant (portion of the night) | 59% | 73% |
| Infant facing mother (portion of the night) | 46% | 65% |
| Face to face (portion of the night) | 32% | 47% |
| **Average Infant Sleep Positions** | | |
| Infant on back (portion of the night) | 83% | 40% |
| Infant on side (portion of the night) | 6% | 54% |
| Infant on tummy (portion of the night) | 0% | 0% |
| **Height of Infant in Bed Relative to Mother** | | |
| Infant face level with mother's face or chin | 71% | 0% |
| Infant face level with mother's chest | 29% | 100% |
| **Average Feeding Frequency** | | |
| Number of bouts (per night) | 1 | 2.5 |
| Total feeding time (per night) | 9 minutes | 31 minutes |
| **Awakening Frequency** | | |
| Maternal arousals (per night) | 0–4 | 3–5 |
| Infant arousals (per night) | 0–3 | 2–5 |
| Mutual arousals (per night) | 0–2 | 1–4 |

Fig. 3.3 A study lead by Dr. Helen Ball compares the behavior and sleep positions that affect nighttime safety for bedsharing mother-infant pairs, based on whether or not the infant is breastfed.

formula- or bottle-feeding mothers tend to place their baby by their face, closer to or on top of pillows that can potentially be a suffocation hazard.[96, 97, 98]

Dr. Ball also noted that breastsleeping mothers and babies tend to arouse more quickly in response to each other's stirrings than non-breastfeeding, bedsharing mothers and babies. My own research also clearly showed this increased sensitivity, even when comparing consistently bedsharing, breastfeeding pairs to other breastfeeding pairs who only bedshare part of the time.[11, 19, 99]

One of our studies found that the average breastfeeding interval of routinely breastsleeping mothers is close to an hour and a half, which is approximately the length of the human sleep cycle.[100] This supports the possibility that the nutritional needs of breastfeeding infants influenced the evolved average length of the human sleep cycle, so that mothers complete their sleep cycles at about the same time their infant needs to be fed again. This speculation could be tested by looking at other mammals, comparing the milk composition and total calories per feed to the characteristics and average length of their adult sleep cycle.

For the same reasons that it is safer for breastfeeding mother-baby pairs to bedshare, it is also best for breastsleeping infants to sleep between the mother and the side of the bed, rather than between the mother and any other adult sharing the sleep surface. Breastsleeping infants do not have the same sensitivities to their non-breastfeeding parent or any other adult who may be in the bed.

The overall physiological and behavioral characteristics that accompany breastsleeping, considered alongside humanity's long history of evolved nighttime care abilities, explain why telling parents to never sleep with their baby is not going to work. If an evolved taste for fats and sugars mirrors our biological drive to bedshare, then trying to stop bedsharing altogether is like suggesting nobody should eat fats and sugars at all. Excessive fats and sugars can lead to obesity or death from heart disease, diabetes, or cancer, but, obviously, there's a whole lot more to the story. Our bodies still need these things to function, and as long as we make careful and thoughtful choices about how we incorporate them into our lives, they can contribute greatly to our overall health and satisfaction.

)

# Why Cosleeping Is Important for Breastfeeding, Bottle-Feeding, and Formula-Feeding

Due to the low-calorie composition of human breastmilk, which is genetically suited to the human infant's underdeveloped gut, infants must nurse frequently around the clock, including at night. Anthropologist Dr. Carol Worthman from Emory University followed breastfeeding Kalahari !Kung Bushmen mothers and

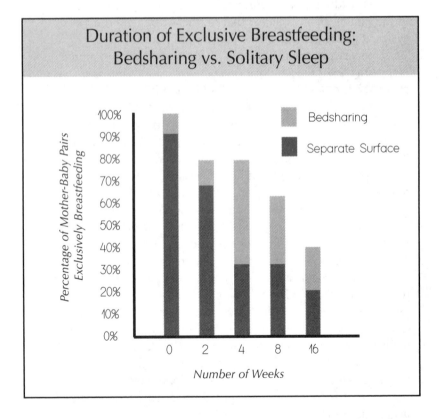

*Fig. 3.4 Dr. Helen Ball's research shows here that, compared with solitary-sleeping mothers, breastsleeping mothers are more likely to breastfeed their infants for a greater number of weeks, and are more likely to meet their breastfeeding goals.*

babies during the day as the women gathered nuts and berries. She found that these carried babies consistently snacked on breastmilk every 13 minutes for a few minutes at a time.[101] While most mothers in Western societies are unable to carry their babies throughout the day, keeping babies close at night can help meet their nutritional and emotional needs.

For those mothers who feel as though they are missing out on essential aspects of motherhood, cosleeping may help counter these concerns. As one parent phrased it to me, spending nights beside her baby helped "validate her role as a loving mother." This may be particularly helpful for parents who spend many daytime hours away from their baby while at work.[16, 36] The fact that U.S. employers offer little to no maternity leave means most American new mothers need to return to work before the recommended time required to meet optimal breastfeeding recommendations. This may explain, in part, what has caused such a cultural shift toward increased cosleeping behavior. Approximately 81% of U.S. mothers leave the hospital breastfeeding, and even mothers who never intended to bedshare soon discover how much easier breastfeeding is, and how much more satisfied they feel with their baby sleeping alongside them.

Our intensive laboratory studies reveal that babies who are breastfed and share a room with their mothers tend to nurse more often, and for longer periods of time, than breastfeeding mothers and infants sleeping in separate rooms.[12]

> Mothers who breastsleep with their infants often report that they hardly need to wake up when the baby is hungry.

Mothers who breastsleep with their infants often report that they hardly need to wake up when the baby is hungry, or that they need only awaken for a few minutes to get the baby latched on. The baby nurses as needed, and mom continues to sleep with subconscious awareness of how the baby is doing.

According to the American Academy of Pediatrics Policy Statement, in the section about breastfeeding, babies should not have to cry in order for caregivers to know they are hungry. The AAP and other lactation scientists

# Can You Breastsleep if You Are Mixed-Feeding?

Mixed-feeding involves giving your infant formula in conjunction with milk directly from your breast, expressed breastmilk (bottled using a breast pump), or donor breastmilk. Although exclusive breastfeeding directly from the breast is the best option for any baby, there are many reasons why a mother may consider mixed-feeding, including health risks, pain, infection, sickness, or insufficient milk supply. Whatever your reason, it is important to point out that the more you breastfeed, the safer your baby is. A baby receiving even a small amount of breastmilk during each feed should be reason to celebrate, and I hope you can feel very good about it. If you are experiencing any complications, consider working with a lactation consultant.

The safety of bedsharing while mixed-feeding is a question that has never been adequately studied, so we have very little data on the matter. My research knowledge leads me to think that partial breastfeeding and exclusive breastfeeding are both linked with a decreased risk of SIDS at all ages. I am not aware of any large-scale, population-based studies that shed light on this issue directly, but you can check out a study from 1998 led by Kathryn G. Dewey for a related perspective.[102] With that in mind, the studies we do have show the risk of SIDS to be halved when breastfeeding is exclusive at one month, but when infants are only partially breastfed, we just don't know yet to what degree bedsharing is a safe option.[103] I would generally recommend bedsharing with your baby only if he or she was exclusively breastfed directly from the breast for the first month of life, but I would not say it is impossible to provide a safe enough environment to breastsleep while mixed-feeding.

If you do bottle-feed part of the time, even if you bottle-feed expressed breastmilk or donor breastmilk, be aware that there may be certain cues established by exclusive, direct breastfeeding that you could still miss. While bottle-fed infants who receive breastmilk may sleep in safer, lighter stages of sleep than formula-fed infants, breastfeeding directly from the breast further affects arousal patterns and sensitivity for both moms and babies.[8] Direct breastfeeding also changes where and how the baby is placed next to the mother,[99] but this information is easy to learn. If you have established exclusive breastfeeding for one month, and are planning to switch to mixed-feeding, I would say it becomes up to you whether you feel it is safe enough to continue breastsleeping.

agree that "crying is a late indicator of hunger."[104] The best way, or perhaps the only way, to know if your baby is hungry before he or she starts crying, is to be close enough to hear the baby's sounds and to feel the baby's wiggles, arm movements, and facial cues, which act as nonverbal invitations to be fed.

A study by Dr. Helen Ball in Great Britain shows that the greater convenience of breastfeeding while bedsharing promotes a greater commitment to breastfeed for a greater number of months, resulting in long-term health benefits for infants and mothers alike.[16]

However, not all mothers choose to or are able to breastfeed. Mothers who feed their babies breastmilk from a bottle instead of from the breast can still offer some immunological protection and health benefits for their babies—and the more breastmilk the baby receives, the better. Any amount of breastmilk is much better than none. While I generally don't recommend bedsharing for bottle-fed infants, roomsharing mothers who bottle-feed their babies with breastmilk still feed their babies more often than separate-sleeping families. This provides the baby with more nutrition, healthy weight gain, and home-grown antibodies.[102, 105]

If a mother is unable to provide breastmilk at all, she should not bedshare, but there are still advantages to roomsharing. These advantages include more frequent instances of formula-feeding, which increases opportunities to check on the baby throughout the night. Roomsharing offers significant added protection against SIDS, regardless of whether the baby is or is not breastfeeding or receiving breastmilk. Although I have to repeat that formula-feeding itself is a risk factor for SIDS, my educated guess is that roomsharing can mitigate—however slightly—the dangers of not breastfeeding.

Beyond the health benefits of increased feeding time, cosleeping is important because both breast and bottle-feeding babies respond positively to being touched and hearing a parent's movements and breathing. They are reassured and physiologically affected by the caregiver's presence. The more parent and infant are in close proximity, the better each becomes at interpreting and responding in kind to each other's signals and cues and the better they communicate. This is especially important to bottle-fed babies who might miss out on some of the frequent contact and intense bonding that takes place during breastfeeding.

What I'm saying is that, regardless of feeding method, all infants can benefit emotionally and psychologically by sensing and reacting to their parent's attention, contact, and proximity. Parents also benefit from this closeness, building stronger attachment to their infant—and vice versa—whether the baby is on a separate surface or the same surface. A number of studies show that attachment and maternal sensitivity, as well as emotional bonding, is improved through increased physical holding and carrying both day and night.[96, 106] This is something that can be achieved through both breastfeeding and formula- or bottle-feeding.[86]

While skin-to-skin contact can occur during periods in which the infant is awake during the night, it is probably best for most families who bottle-feed (with breastmilk, formula, or a mix of the two) to cosleep by placing the infant next to the bed on a different surface, rather than in the bed. However, as always, you are in the best position to judge exactly how sensitive and responsive you can be to your baby. Ideally, you could discuss this decision with an informed, objective pediatrician who is willing to consider your personal values before giving a recommendation. For now, this seems sadly unlikely given the contentious nature of the bedsharing debate, and the awkward position pediatricians find themselves in if they disagree with the AAP.

## Bedsharing for Fathers

Humans are one of the few species of mammals in which fathers are heavily invested in their children and help mothers in taking care of them. In fact, only 5% of all mammals have males that participate either directly or indirectly in the care of their offspring.[107] Because males are generally not considered the primary caregiver in the mammalian world, including in traditional Western family structures, little attention has been paid to what fathers might contribute to the care of their infants in a bedsharing context, with the majority of attention focused on the mother-infant relationship. Even less is known about a father's capacity to be responsive in ways similar to a breastsleeping mother.

However, Dr. Lee T. Gettler, my colleague at the University of Notre Dame, published a paper that characterized the uniqueness of evolved human male reproductive physiology in comparison to most other primate males, describing in what way fathers might have come to play an important role in contributing to the survival and well-being of their offspring.

Historically, men helping to carry their infants could have reduced the high demands placed on mothers, which in turn could have helped reduce the inter-birth interval. This may be what made it possible for families to support two completely dependent offspring at a time, a unique human adaptation.[108]

After this research, Dr. Gettler and his colleagues went on to produce a series of empirical papers [100, 108, 109, 110, 111, 112, 113] that extensively examined changes in human male neuroendocrinology. Specifically, they studied changes in hormone levels as men move

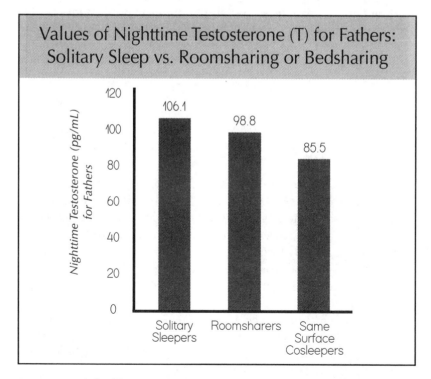

*Fig. 3.5 A study lead by Dr. Lee T. Gettler (and myself) shows low levels of nighttime testosterone in fathers who bedshare, which may promote better childcare practices.*

from dating, to partnering with a woman, to having their first child and spending time playing or bedsharing with them.

They first demonstrated that, as human males transition from a single or dating reproductive status to partnering with a woman, their testosterone significantly declines,[113] just as it does when they become fathers,[109] and when they spend more time playing with their children.[110, 112, 113]

At this point, multiple studies have found that engaged fathers have lower levels of testosterone than unpartnered, childless males.[100] Cross-species data shows that high testosterone can and often does interfere with paternal investment, leading to lower offspring growth and reduced survival. Evidence from studies of the behavior and socioendocrinology of human males suggests that men with lower testosterone are likely more sensitive and responsive to children's needs. Lower testosterone levels could improve daytime father-based care as well as nighttime cosleeping, aiding fathers' responses to their children in both instances, which contributes to better child health and development.[106, 113]

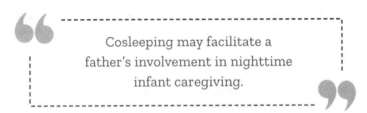

> Cosleeping may facilitate a father's involvement in nighttime infant caregiving.

A study of fathers in Metro Cebu, Philippines, conducted in 2011 and led by Dr. Gettler, found that fathers who slept near their children on the same surface had greater declines in testosterone during the day and lower evening levels compared to fathers who slept separately from their children.[100] These results were the first to show that testosterone is comparatively lower among fathers practicing bedsharing compared to solitary-sleeping fathers, and suggests that cosleeping may cause testosterone levels to decline and remain relatively low. The findings also suggest that bedsharing fathers may maintain lower testosterone once children move out of infancy and become toddlers and beyond, while for solitary-sleeping fathers, it may increase.

The experience of sleeping with their infant can also help relieve some of the distancing effects felt by fathers, who are

# Should I Bedshare if My Partner Is Not the Baby's Father?

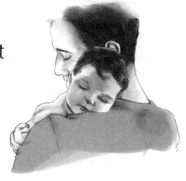

There is at least one study that has shown an increased risk of an infant dying when bedsharing with an unrelated adult in the bed. The study was called the Chicago Infant Mortality Study, conducted by Dr. Fern Hauck. The study came to the conclusion that "bedsharing was only a risk when the infant was sleeping with people other than the parents."[46] However, the group that was studied showed multiple other risk factors present for many of the infant deaths.

Here are some further thoughts. If an unrelated sleeping partner considers the breastsleeping infant their responsibility in the same way that the mother does, then breastsleeping should be as safe as it would be if the biological father or an adoptive parent were bedsharing. When trying to determine this, the important issues to wrestle with include what kind of relationship this partner, male or female, has with both the mother and the infant, how much the act of bedsharing means to them, and to what degree they accept responsibility for the infant's safety. In this situation, it may be best to err on the side of caution by keeping the baby on a separate surface next to the bed, or only placing the infant in the bed when the mother is breastfeeding. Should you choose to bedshare, it is likely that the baby would be safer sleeping next to the mother only, and not in between both parents. Yet again, more research on this topic is desperately needed. As it stands, there is no simple yes or no answer to the question of whether it is safe.

Certainly, both commitment and the degree of protection that a person feels for an infant changes how the adult sleeps, affecting their arousals so they can adequately respond to the infant's needs. Breastfeeding makes this more effective for mothers, but that does not mean that a loving, committed partner cannot exhibit vigilance during sleep if they decide to do so, and if they are emotionally invested in the infant's health and well-being.

However, to be explicit, unrelated adults might not feel responsibility for the infant's safety in the same way as a biological or adoptive parent. This is understandable, but in any situation where this is true, I would definitely recommend against any bedsharing. Instead, place the baby next to the bed on a separate surface.

outside of the breastfeeding relationship. Cosleeping may facilitate a father's involvement in nighttime infant caregiving.[106, 113] If bedsharing, both parents should agree and feel comfortable with the decision. Each bedsharer should agree that he or she is equally responsible for the infant, and should acknowledge that they are aware the infant is present in the bed space. As stated previously, in most cases, the baby should only sleep next to the breastfeeding mother, not in between both adults.

Admittedly, I could never say with confidence that any father who is the primary caregiver could not train himself, like the mother, to be acceptably sensitive to the infant. This is another good example of a question that has never been fully explored. We likely won't receive an answer until governmental and civic organizations decide to allocate research funds toward bedsharing safety.

As far as I can tell, only two studies to date[15, 99] have offered any specific information on behavior of fathers in a bedsharing context. But we do have some preliminary data from a small study I conducted alongside Dr. Gettler and our undergraduate student, Michael Paluzzi. This study, presented in 2013, used infrared recordings of the interactions between mom, dad, and baby while sleeping in the same bed. The study focused on similarities and differences in waking patterns, length of time spent in contact with the infant, and body orientations of participating mothers and fathers.

After reviewing ten-minute recordings taken every hour throughout the night, we were somewhat surprised by what we found. Fathers and mothers displayed similar arousal patterns in response to their infants. A father would usually respond after the mother had done so first, often raising his head to look over at what was going on with the baby, placing his arm over the mother to reach the baby, or briefly touching the mother or infant with transient brushes of his hand.

If supported by future studies, these results may be used to help us understand how these important nighttime exchanges between fathers and their infants potentially influence each other's underlying physiologies,[108] possibly facilitating more nurturing care or patience with their babies in fathers who bedshare.

Fathers did not, however, spend as much time in physical contact with their infants, especially compared to breastfeeding mothers. In general, we observed that mothers were in contact with their infants for an average of 56% of the observations, and fathers were only in contact with their infants for about 12% of the time recorded.

They also did not face their infants as much throughout the night. While fathers were oriented toward their infants 41% of the time—a meaningful percentage of our observations—mothers faced their infants much more frequently at 73%.

Speaking of what fathers do or don't do while sleeping with their babies, a student of Dr. Helen Ball also conducted a small study on the matter. For his master's thesis at Durham University of Great Britain, Steve Leech studied both fathers and mothers sleeping with infants up to 12 weeks old.[114] For three consecutive nights, the infants alternated randomly between bedsharing and sleeping on a separate surface next to the bed in a cot or crib. Leech monitored and recorded each infant's temperature, breathing rate, and oxygen saturation levels (percentage of oxygen in the infant's blood) throughout each night. Mothers and fathers also wore monitors to record breathing rate and oxygen levels. Infrared cameras placed above the sleepers filmed all of their nighttime behavior.

Based mainly on movement patterns, Leech was able to roughly identify when each person was awake, experiencing REM sleep, or experiencing the other stages of sleep, collectively called NREM (Non-Rapid Eye Movement) or quiet sleep. In my own studies, more full polysomnography (recording of brain waves, oxygen levels, heart rate, and eye and body movements) could distinguish the sleep stages within NREM, such as Stages 1–2 (light sleep) and Stages 3–4 (deep sleep).[97]

In this small study, breastfeeding and bedsharing mothers exhibited less time awake on the bedsharing nights than when the infants slept next to them in a cot, while infants spent less time in quiet sleep on the bedsharing night. Regularly bedsharing infants seemed to experience more disruption or fragmentation of their usual sleep when sleeping in the cot than when they slept snuggled up to their mothers in bed.

Regardless of whether the father was in the bed or not, mothers exhibited a higher degree of sleep state synchrony, meaning mother and baby shared more time in the same sleep status (awake, in REM sleep, or in quiet sleep) when the infant was in the bed instead of in the cot. Moreover, both mothers and infants exhibited more arousals overall, and shared more partner-induced arousals, when the baby was bedsharing, findings that are in agreement with our more detailed physiological studies.[97]

In contrast, no sleep stage synchrony was found between dad and baby when the baby was sleeping in the bed or by the bed, and regardless of whether they were regular bedsharers or regular beside-the-bed cosleepers. Unlike in our own small study of fathers here in the U.S., paternal arousal in this study was entirely unaffected by the location of the infant. But, interestingly, fathers' absence from the bed did seem to have an effect. While fathers were absent, infants experienced more awakenings and less REM, while a few mothers experienced less REM, and one mother experienced less waking time but more REM and more overall sleep.

It is hard to explain why the American dads in my 2013 study with Dr. Gettler seemed to be more aware of what was going on in the bed, with increased arousal time and engagement with their infants that is not seen in Leech's study. However, it would be irresponsible to draw firm conclusions from either study because the sample sizes are very small.

It might be noted that a poll taken in Great Britain and published in *Sleep Health* in 2004 found that half of the polled dads, whether routinely or irregularly bedsharing, admitted to pretending to be asleep to avoid nighttime caregiving. Something tells me that there may well be a cultural difference operating here, which affects paternal responsivity to cosleeping infants in Great Britain versus the United States, but I will leave it to the mothers from our two respective societies to decide if this possibility is plausible.

Having said all of that, it is hard for me to tell other men that you simply cannot exhibit the same degree of sensitivity as a breastsleeping mother. I am sure that even my wife would take issue with that statement, after watching my responsive behavior with our infant son in 1978. When he would awaken and want to breastfeed, I was usually the one to immediately wake up, take him out of his bassinet next to our bed, and get him set up to breastfeed, then put him back when he was finished. Keep in mind that, at this point, I had not done the research on bedsharing—nor had anyone else—so we were only breastsleeping episodically. If we had known what we know now, we certainly would have had our son in bed with us more consistently.

It is worth reminding you that, aside from never letting an infant sleep outside the presence of a committed adult, until they are at least 6–12 months old, I do not recommend to anyone specifically whether they should bedshare, breastsleep, or cosleep in some other form. Where a baby sleeps reflects who we are, our personalities, our individual histories, our access to resources, our emotions, and our own needs. I do not know the particular circumstances of each family, how much they know about safety precautions, or what bedsharing means to them. What I do recommend is to consider all of the possible choices and to become as informed as possible, matching what you learn with what you think will work the best for you, your baby, and your family.[115, 116]

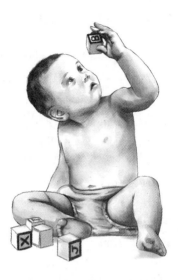

CHAPTER 7

# Benefits of Cosleeping

## The Positive Effects of Breastfeeding

We know that breastsleeping and even roomsharing tends to increase the frequency and duration of breastfeeding, but what makes that so important? To start with, breastfeeding provides the opportunity for your newborn to learn and practice communicative cues. These cues create a bond between you and your baby that can better protect them through arousals while you bedshare at night.

This is part of the reason why bedsharing is most safely practiced by breastfeeding mother-baby pairs—because they are conditioned to respond to each other's arousals. Mothers who exclusively breastfeed also position their sleeping baby close to their chest, a safer alternative when compared to mothers who formula-or mixed-feed, who tend to place their baby close to their face while bedsharing.

Babies are also generally happier and more willing to engage with their environments when they are breastfed by their mothers.[117]

# Benefits of Breastsleeping for Babies

- **Greater breastmilk supply**

  As babies breastfeed throughout the night, their suckling stimulates their mothers to create more of the milk needed for proper nourishment.

- **More frequent breastfeeding**

  Studies tell us that more frequent feeds reduce time spent crying, thereby contributing to your baby's energy conservation and calm wakefulness.

- **Longer breastfeeding sessions**

  Longer feedings ensure that your baby receives enough calories daily to provide adequate nutrition and weight gain.

- **Longer breastfeeding period**

  By continually breastfeeding over time, babies receive the immunological and nutritional benefits they need for optimum growth and development.

- **Increased safety**

  Breastfeeding babies, as opposed to formula-fed, are being constantly monitored throughout the night, and tend to be placed on their backs, in the recommended supine position, with their noses and mouths unobstructed.

- **Increased infant sleep duration**

  Babies who sleep alone must cry loudly and long enough to wake their parents who are sleeping several rooms away. By sleeping together, babies achieve a longer and better rest period.

- **Lower stress levels**

  When babies do not have to cry, thus becoming agitated, to have their needs met, they are able to stay calmer and more content.

- **Temperature regulation**

  Babies are warmer when they sleep next to their moms, and mothers can sense their baby's temperature and respond by adding a blanket if her infant seems chilled, or by removing covers if her infant is overheated.

- **Increased sensitivity to mother's communication**

  Moms and babies who routinely sleep together have a heightened and enhanced sensitivity to each other's smells, movements, and touches.

*Fig. 3.6 Combined breastfeeding and bedsharing provides many benefits for infants.*

Biologically speaking, of course there is more to breastmilk than just building connections and being happy. Breastmilk is the primary and best architect of the infant's developing brain, and maybe this is why breastfed babies score higher on IQ tests and other cognitive tests than formula-fed babies.[117]

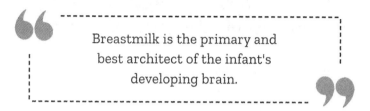

> Breastmilk is the primary and best architect of the infant's developing brain.

Exciting new neurobiological research on the developing human infant's brain has shown that breastmilk increases the density of "white matter," or brain cells that facilitate cell to cell (neuron to neuron) communication.[118]

One large-scale study comparing breast, mixed-, and bottle-feeding infants' weight gain showed that higher (meaning healthier) weight gain in the first few months was associated with more frequent breastfeeding.[105]

Breastmilk also contains immunoglobulin and cytokines, which help stave off infections that are believed to contribute to SIDS.[103] Multiple studies reveal that more breastfeeding translates to more protection from SIDS.[12, 99, 105] This is why the American Academy of Pediatrics now recommends breastfeeding as a preventative measure against many conditions and diseases.

Frequent breastfeeding ensures that infants receive greater immunological benefits than infants who are exclusively or primarily formula-fed. The more often babies nurse, and the more breastmilk they are given, the more antibodies they receive. These are designer antibodies, produced by the mother specifically to fight bacteria found in the infant's own home environment and any viruses or bacteria to which the mother and baby are exposed. For newborns, who are particularly vulnerable to disease because of their immature immune systems, these antibodies can provide vital protection from dangerous, fast-acting, and potentially fatal infectious diseases.[102]

Until relatively recently, we had no scientific evidence regarding how many infant lives breastfeeding might save in industrialized

nations. Even in a country like the United States, where
infectious diseases are largely under control due to our strict
sanitary practices, a recent epidemiological study showed that

## Benefits of Separate-Surface Cosleeping for the Formula-Fed Baby and Parents

- **Nurturing sleep environment**

  Mothers and fathers who sleep close by their babies are able to
  respond quickly if their infant cries, chokes, needs their nasal passages
  cleared, needs to be cooled or warmed, or simply needs to be held.
  Cosleeping babies are more confident that their needs will be met
  almost immediately.

- **Emotionally reassuring**

  Babies who sleep with their parents receive the comfort of their
  mothers' and fathers' touch, warmth, and protection. For parents
  who work outside the home, separate-surface cosleeping can be a
  wonderfully restorative time to reconnect with their baby.

- **Safety**

  Depending on the degree of the mother's desire to sleep in contact
  with her infant, and her capacity or ability to sustain a safe sleep
  environment, side-by-side cosleeping (on different surfaces) and
  roomsharing (rather than bedsharing) may well be the safest and most
  reassuring way to cosleep for the bottle-feeding mother-infant pair.

- **Lower stress**

  A parent's presence can be extremely reassuring to babies if they are ill
  or irritable, and being able to immediately monitor the baby's state can
  provide parents with peace of mind throughout the night.

- **More sleep**

  Separate-surface cosleeping babies cry less frequently and sleep more
  often than solitary-sleeping babies, and you can meet his or her needs
  without having to leave your room and walk to the crib, saving you
  time as well.

*Fig. 3.7 If your infant is not breastfed, it is not as safe to bedshare. However, there are still many benefits to separate-surface cosleeping.*

approximately 720 American babies die each year from congenital or infectious diseases, or illness complications, because they were not fed breastmilk.[61] This study clearly demonstrates that, even in a highly industrialized Western culture, the number of infant lives saved by breastfeeding is impressive.

## Nighttime Contact Is Good for Babies

A baby who sleeps in proximity to his or her parents, whether bedsharing or sleeping on a separate surface, benefits from the continual reminders of the caregivers' presence—inspections, touches, smells, movement, warmth, and, by virtue of increased breastfeeding, taste. These sensations provide emotional security for the baby.

Studying infants in New Zealand, Dr. Sally Baddock's team found that bedsharing infants were touched by their mothers, rather than just looked at, almost three times more often during the night than solitary-sleeping infants, with an average of eleven physical inspections each night, compared to only four.[15]

Both preterm and full-term infants can benefit significantly just from the physical presence of their parents. Cosleeping children are significantly more likely to have a secure attachment to their parents, compared to solitary sleepers,[119] and roomsharing infants learn at a faster rate due to the greater number of social interactions and frequent communication that comes with increased contact and proximity. Scientific studies show that when babies rest on their mothers' or fathers' chest, enjoying direct skin-to-skin contact, they breathe more regularly, use energy more efficiently, grow faster, and experience less stress.[120]

Research in the early 2000s by Drs. Sari Goldstein, Imad Makhoul, and Helen Ball pointed out that skin-to-skin contact, referred to as kangaroo care, leads to earlier discharge of premature infants from the NICU, fewer apneas, and fewer bradycardia incidents (periods of slow heart rates).[105, 121] A recent meta-analysis, combining many studies, revealed that skin-to-skin kangaroo care reduced mortality among preterm infants by as much as 36%, while leading to increased head circumference, higher oxygenation levels, decreased numbers of sepsis cases, less hypoglycemia, and fewer readmissions to the hospital.[47, 122]

A now-classic 2005 study by Dr. Jan Winberg also showed that skin-to-skin contact with the mother immediately after birth regulated infants' temperature, eliminating the need for an incubator. Moreover, infants who experienced skin-to-skin contact showed better energy storage and higher blood sugar levels compared with babies being warmed in an incubator.[123] Relatedly, a separate study found that preterm infants enjoying skin-to-skin care retained their core body temperature for hours, and maternal breast temperature matched the infants' core temperature needs.[124]

Maternal contact is known to act as a painkiller for babies, and increased touching and holding helps newborns recover rapidly from birth-related fatigue.[125] Physical contact also facilitates spontaneous breastfeeding and encourages mothers to breastfeed for longer periods of time per breastfeeding session.[126] Infants who experience skin-to-skin care sleep for longer periods and seem less agitated in general. Close contact also helps them enjoy more stable heart rates and breathing patterns, leading to greater overall oxygenation.[127]

Skin-to-skin contact is associated with a significant increase in maternal oxytocin levels (a hormone released during breastfeeding and social bonding), as described in two Swedish studies.[128] This suggests that uterine contraction would be enhanced and milk ejection improved, to the benefit of both mother and infant. There is a report that skin-to-skin contact is also associated with lowered maternal anxiety and more efficient participation of mothers in caring for their newborn infants.[129]

Other than promoting skin-to-skin contact, cosleeping can also provide a more protected and nurturing nighttime environment. If your baby's well-being is threatened while cosleeping—for example, the infant is choking or struggling to move a blanket away from his or her face—you will (if attentive) be able to help right away (see Appendix IV for examples of potential life-saving responses by bedsharing families). Your baby also benefits from an immediate response to his or her needs.

When babies do not have their needs met, especially before they can verbalize their needs, they cry. Crying evolved as an alarm signal, and is the ultimate way babies communicate their needs. This response is reserved for critical circumstances involving pain, hunger, or fear, and it is used to elicit mothers' retrieval behavior. It is a well-known fact that crying decreases oxygenation and increases heart rate, which in turn augments cortisol, a stress hormone.

Some studies suggest that chronic elevated levels of cortisol in infancy can cause physical changes in the brain, promoting a greater vulnerability to social attachment disorders.[86, 96] At the very least, the energy lost in crying could be better put into growth or maintenance.[130] Babies who breastsleep or roomshare are much less likely to cry themselves to sleep, or even cry at all, and so avoid releasing an excess of this hormone.

However, many parents are now encouraged to use "controlled crying techniques" to manage infants and young children who do not settle alone, who wake at night, or who settle only if held or permitted to sleep in proximity with the parents. So concerned is the Australian Association of Infant Mental Health about the use of such techniques that they issued the following statement: "...controlled crying is not consistent with what infants need for their optimal emotional and psychological health, and may have unintended negative consequences."[131]

> My wife and I let my infant son cry it out for about 15 minutes. It remains the only 15 minutes of my life I wish I could take back.

Letting babies cry themselves to sleep is advice given to parents with the goal of raising children that are self-reliant, able to comfort themselves, and comfortable with aloneness. The entire idea is a social construct. Cosleeping children do tend to sleep through the night at a later age than enforced solitary-sleeping babies—about a year to a year and a half later—but all children will eventually be able to wake up and fall asleep again by themselves. Sleep training offers no actual advantage, and the most careful research completed thus far actually leads to the opposite conclusion.

Several studies show that bottle-fed, enforced solitary-sleeping babies experience more consolidated sleep. One study compared development of sleep between infants who experienced minimal bottle-feeding and contact during the night—recommended by Dr. Benjamin Spock—and infants who experienced prolonged breastfeeding and physical contact, as encouraged by the breastfeeding support organization La Leche League.[132]

Among bottle-feeding infants receiving minimal nighttime contact, the average length of sleeping bouts increased from six-and-a-half hours at two months of age to eight hours at four months, and to greater than eight hours during the second year.

In contrast to the consolidated sleep of the Spock-care infants, the sleep of breastfed and potentially cosleeping infants was characterized by shorter bouts of sleep and frequent awakenings. At two months of age, these infants slept an average of only five hours at a time during their longest sleeping bout. Minimal-contact infants were sleeping up to eight hours by four months, but the high-contact infants did not sleep significantly longer than five hours until they were 20 months old.

Total nightly sleep time also developed differently for contact sleepers. La Leche League infants slept a total of 15 hours at two months, 12.5 hours at four months, and just over 11 hours by two years. Spock-care infants continued to sleep 13–14 hours per day throughout the two-year monitoring period.[132, 133] The study concluded that feeding choices and sleep contact have major effects on the development of sleep patterns.

But, I repeat, all children will come to exhibit longer sleep bouts in relationship to the family's general patterns. No infant needs to be sleep trained. I confess to having strong feelings about this based on a personal experience. When I was a young parent, before I knew what I know today, my wife and I let my infant son cry it out for about 15 minutes. It remains the only 15 minutes of my life I wish I could take back. It was like torture for my little son, and his feelings of suffering and rejection were completely unwarranted. When I opened the door, he was standing at his crib rail, eyes swollen, sobbing and hyperventilating. I saw only love and relief in his face at seeing me, and my own heart broke.

Because of that personal experience, I get upset that anyone in authority would suggest that this is okay and in the baby's best interest. It isn't. Based on studies of psychologically-injured children and adults, researchers are now finding that leaving children to cry without offering any comfort may cause, in extreme cases, lasting damage to their brains. We have no idea yet what changes might occur at the level of the DNA itself.

## New Discoveries on the Lasting Effects of Close Contact

For mammal babies, and especially for those less mature at birth (like humans), early experiences and deprivation of maternal contact and proximity can actually influence the activity of their genes, potentially affecting psychological resilience, metabolism, and immune functionality. This happens through a process called methylation. Changes in the DNA occur when carbon and hydrogen are added to the genes, like "dimmer switches" turning on and off, affecting infant behavior and physiology. One major surprise is that these immediate changes to genetic activity may also be passed on to following generations.

> There can be significant, genetically-driven behavioral consequences in humans due to the quality of care they receive as an infant. This change in the gene can even be passed on to future generations.

A famous experiment on rat pups, led by Dr. Michael Meany, showed that greater nurturing in the form of more breastfeeding, licking, and grooming by mother rats led the offspring to experience less anxiety and fear when confronting stressful situations. Researchers at Brown University, led by Dr. Barry M. Lester, recently hypothesized that we might expect similar results for humans.[5]

Dr. Lester wanted to examine the gene sites that regulate an infant's stress reactions, specifically the gluco-corticoid receptor gene in charge of fluctuations in cortisol. Exclusively-breastfed infants experience more contact with their mothers and receive more health benefits from breastmilk than formula- or mixed-fed infants, so Dr. Lester's research team theorized that more alterations in the relevant gene, through the process of DNA-methylation, would be found in the formula- or mixed-fed babies—called "low-contact" infants. They hypothesized that fewer alterations would be found in the "high-contact," exclusively-breastfeeding infants, who would exhibit, like the highly-nurtured rat pups, less stress response when presented with a stressful challenge.

Using small samples of cheek tissue and saliva, the infant's cortisol levels and changes in molecular structure were measured before and after a stress-inducing experiment. The stress test they used was a well-known procedure called the "still-face." In this test, a mother spends two minutes joyously engaging with her infant, face-to-face. For the next two minutes, she suddenly stops any expression and stares at her infant without smiling or showing positive emotion. The infant then tries to "win" the mother back. Upon failing to do so, the baby normally shows great distress and sadness, with some infants drooling or hiccupping, stretching out while crying, and looking away.

The authors of the DNA study point out that the response by the exclusively-breastfed human infants mirrored the results from the experiment done on the rats. It seemed that the maternal nurturing behaviors had a specific effect on the DNA, making the low-contact infants react more severely to the still-face test than the high-contact infants. The DNA analysis showed different gluco-corticoid receptor genes present in the low-contact babies compared to the high-contact babies, due to the methylation process. The researchers concluded that variations in maternal care alter the underlying genome of the infant, which, in turn, alters stress reactivity.

The implication is that there can be significant, genetically-driven behavioral consequences in humans and other mammals due to the nature and quality of care they receive as an infant. Such changes in gene sites may potentially be passed on to future generations, but much research is needed to verify for how many genomic sites this could be true, or under what biological circumstances this happens.

In a similar recent study, led by Dr. Sarah R. Moore, parents of five-week-old babies kept a diary of their infants' behaviors (such as sleeping, fussing, crying, or feeding) as well as the duration of caregiving that involved bodily contact. After analyzing DNA samples from each infant, similar to Dr. Lester's study, the researchers concluded that the amount of holding and close comforting infants receive—the exact kind of stimulation that breastsleeping provides—can have a positive effect at the molecular level.[134]

It is the first study of its kind to show so clearly that the need for infant contact with a caregiver is deeply rooted and has potentially life-long consequences on genetic expressions. Researchers found consistent differences in gene activities (by way of the same methylation process) when comparing between high-contact and low-contact children at five specific DNA sites.[135] One of these sites plays a role in the immune system, and another in calibrating metabolism. A press release by the University of British Columbia, where the research was conducted, suggests that "the children who experienced higher distress and received relatively little contact had an 'epigenetic age' that was lower than would be expected, given their actual age." In other studies, a low epigenetic age is linked with poor health outcomes.[136]

In another, very different line of neuro-biological research, new remarkable insights have been uncovered by investigators at the University of California, San Francisco. The team, led by Dr. Mercedes F. Paredes, studied how the neuro-architecture of the human infant's brain develops. They found something completely unexpected and possibly unique to human beings. The momentous research paper, published in 2016,[18] has major implications for how early experiences such as breastsleeping could play a role in shaping an infant's neurological development, potentially reducing susceptibilities to future mental or physical disorders.

The researchers found a previously undiscovered mass of thousands of young, undeveloped nerve cells lined up in an arc behind the human infant's eyes. On the first day of life, up to about three months of age, these young neurons embark on a migratory journey on their way to the prefrontal cortex, located roughly behind the infant's forehead. The prefrontal cortex is the center of cognition, and makes possible what is called "executive functioning," which refers to more complex thinking like judgments, evaluations, stop-go activities, discrimination, and general problem solving.

According to this study, what those young neurons will become and where they end up in the brain seem to be influenced by what the infant is experiencing in his or her environment. This includes all types of sensory and intellectual stimulation as well as social interactions provided by caregivers. These unformed nerve cells actually differentiate into various types of nerve cells during their journey depending on what the infant experiences, including being held, touched, spoken to, and played with. Face to face interactions build what some call a "neurological scaffolding," or a foundation for intelligence and resilience potentially helping to guard against the development of mental disorders.[134] More contact with the mother's body can make this neurological scaffolding more stable and effective, providing a strong base for the infant's rapidly growing cognitive and emotional functions.[19]

Again, while not part of their research, we know that skin-to-skin contact, increased

> Skin-to-skin contact, increased holding, and general interaction between parent and infant naturally occurs while cosleeping.

holding, and general interaction between parent and infant naturally occur while cosleeping, especially while breastsleeping, with these practices providing more opportunity to gain the many associated benefits. In this way, cosleeping should theoretically contribute to an infant's neurological architecture, changing the types of neurons that form, how many neurons are retained, and where they end up in the pre-frontal cortex.

These new discoveries leave us with much to learn, but we know that recent studies are sounding a warning against contact deprivation and withholding of species-specific care. Lack of contact throughout both day and night—a problem which infants cannot protect themselves against—may have unintended, irreversible consequences that can be inter-generational.

## Breastsleeping and Colic:
## A New Theory About Inconsolable Crying

From around one month to seven months of age, infants learn how to consciously control their breathing in relation to their intended vocalizations. Rather than simply breathing and vocalizing reflexively, infants learn how to manipulate air volume, air release speed, and holding air back—manipulations that will be required for speech later on.

An infant's respiratory system may be less stable during the period of about 4–14 weeks, when human infants are most susceptible to both SIDS and inconsolable crying, known as colic. This is the period in which control over voice and breath begins to develop, as higher- and lower-brain breathing mechanisms merge. The brainstem connects with higher cortical structures, including those that regulate the ratio of oxygen to carbon dioxide, through

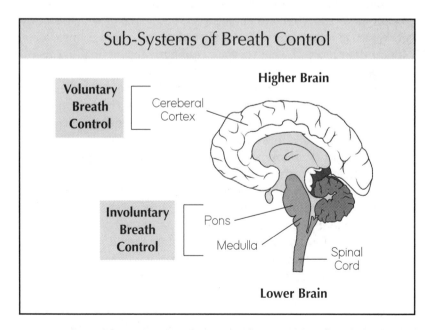

*Fig. 3.8 Colic, and some instances of SIDS, may be caused by infants lacking control over their breathing while voluntary and involuntary sub-systems integrate and develop.*

the growing integration of complex neural pathways. Before this system is mastered and all neurological structures are integrated as they should be, there is room for instabilities where breathing control glitches are possible, giving rise either to SIDS (while asleep) or colic (while awake). My colleagues and I developed a new testable model that looks at what these two prevalent infant health problems have in common.[137]

Humans have two sub-systems of breath control—voluntary and involuntary—and an infant must learn to use both at the same time. The sub-systems are controlled by two different types of neurons in the infant's brain. Excitatory neurons allow the infant to initiate a cry and sustain the air underlying it. Inhibitory neurons allow the infant to stop a cry.

The two sub-systems of breath control (one brainstem-based and the other cortical-based) may develop somewhat asynchronously during the process of becoming functionally one system. An infant may lack inhibitory neurons as compared to excitatory neurons before their voluntary and involuntary nerve tracts become fully interconnected.

We propose that inconsolable crying can be explained by an infant having the ability to initiate a cry, but not being able to stop it. When an infant realizes he or she is unable to stop crying, the infant does more of what they are trying to stop: crying. In this way, the infant becomes caught in a cruel loop.

Inconsolable crying may represent the infant being unable to separate their voice (voluntary) from their breath (involuntary), with the two becoming locked, leading to long, continuous cries outside the control of the infant. I would theorize that equalizing the number of excitatory and inhibitory neurons through stimulation and practice is how babies eventually overcome colic.

The other half of this model speculates that SIDS may be the result of the infant transitioning into or out of REM sleep (Rapid Eye Movement, which occurs while dreaming; refer to Chapter 6 for more information on this). The infant would normally switch from involuntary to a combination of both involuntary and voluntary breathing while transitioning into REM, or "active," sleep. Being unable to enter into or out of one of these two breathing control systems means the baby may get stuck between them, and effectively stop breathing. Unable to get enough oxygen, the baby can tragically die from SIDS.[137]

If only we knew of an easy, natural way for babies to improve or speed up their breathing control... breastsleeping, perhaps? It is likely we can't prevent colic or SIDS, but the diversity of sensory exchanges and experiences in a breastsleeping environment might lessen the lack of synchrony between the sub-systems, or accelerate the developmental process toward more efficient breathing control and integration of voluntary and involuntary neural networks.

Touching and sensory engagements with a caregiver provide opportunities for infants to advance a variety of learned social and physical skills, including breath control. Recall how sensitive infants are to breathing cues, like the "breathing" teddy bears from Chapter 6. Touching, hearing breathing sounds, and hearing parents breathe in relation to speech help infants make a smooth developmental transition. Such engagements may help the infant better control their breathing in relationship to the sounds they want to make, including how they want to cry.

> "Breastsleeping may stimulate development of your infant's breathing control."

A study done in 1985 found that six-week-old infants cried and fussed 43% less when they received supplemental carrying. The experiment's conductors hypothesized that the relative lack of infant carrying in modern Western society may predispose infants to colic.[138] It is thought that prolonged bouts of crying characterize the behavior of babies under the caretaking conditions typical in Western societies. Specifically, it is believed that caregiving practices affect the length of crying bouts, rather than the frequency or pattern of the cries.

In a study headed by child health and development researcher Dr. Ronald G. Barr, members of the !Kung bushmen, or !Kung San, were observed for the crying behavior of their infants. They found that, because infants were almost constantly carried and breastfed throughout the day, they cried significantly less than babies in more industrialized societies. The study concludes, "The peak pattern in the !Kung San infants further increases the evidence that caregiving specifically affects duration of crying. The increased carrying [of !Kung infants]...substantially reduced over-all duration."[139]

Necessary sensory engagements all occur while breastsleeping. If you can't constantly carry your baby with you during the day like the !Kung San, it is safe to say that breastsleeping or other forms of cosleeping may stimulate development of your infant's breathing control to help avoid, resolve, or at the very least ease the symptoms of colic, as well as help prevent the much worse tragedy of SIDS.

I should like to add that, while my hypothesis on SIDS and colic reflects some of the available evidence on physiological control mechanisms, also of great importance (or closely linked) are circulatory control mechanisms. By this I mean control over blood pressure and thermoregulation. For humans, circulatory control may be more effective and active in REM sleep than in non-REM sleep, thus the transition between the two may be just as important or complication-inducing as it is for breathing control. Dr. Peter J. Fleming once pointed out to me that, considering the findings of Dr. Christian F. Poets[140] and research led by Dr. Robert G. Meny,[141] unexpected infant deaths actually seem to be more consistent with a failure of circulatory control or its integrative role alongside, or in relation to, respiratory control. In any case, as some of Dr. Fleming's laboratory studies and studies of bedsharing babies in Mongolia seem to suggest, circulatory control during this sleep-stage transition may be more effective for infants when bedsharing than when sleeping alone.[142, 143, 144, 145]

---------------- ❱ ----------------

## How Parents Can Benefit From Breastsleeping

Keep in mind that when we talk about benefits, we are always talking about instances of elective bedsharing, when it is being done safely and the parents are choosing to breastsleep for emotional and relational reasons. There are now several different studies[16, 127, 146] focusing on why parents choose to cosleep. It appears that a myriad of reasons exist for doing so, including the fact that *it just feels right.*

## Benefits of Breastsleeping for Mothers

- **Greater breastmilk supply**

  Breastfeeding on demand throughout the night helps mothers establish and maintain their milk supply.

- **Increased protection from breast and other reproductive cancers**

  Bedsharing increases both breastfeeding frequency and duration in months, increasing the cancer-protective effects of long-term breastfeeding.

- **More rapid excess weight loss after pregnancy**

- **Enhanced attachment and parental fulfillment**

  Especially for working parents, increased time with baby during the night enhances attachment and helps them feel fulfilled as parents.

- **Reassurance that baby is safe**

  Most breastfeeding mothers who routinely bedshare with their babies tend to place their babies on their backs and sleep in a position that keeps the baby from burrowing under pillows or quilts.

- **Increased sleep duration for mother**

  Studies have demonstrated that mothers who sleep with their babies have more sleep and evaluate their sleep more positively than mothers who sleep apart from their infants.

- **Lower stress levels**

  The increased nipple contact that occurs during nocturnal breastfeeds works to increase the mother's production of oxytocin, a hormone that contributes to a sense of calm and well-being.

- **Increased sensitivity to baby's communication**

  Mothers are able to respond quickly if an infant wants to feed, thus lowering anxiety that the baby's needs are not being met.

*Fig. 3.9 Breastsleeping has numerous benefits for babies, but the combination of breastfeeding and cosleeping can also have suprising benefits for moms.*

A cross-cultural survey of over 200 families from the U.S., Great Britain, France, Canada, Australia, and New Zealand revealed that the fear of not reaching babies fast enough during an earthquake or fire, fear of SIDS, fear of the sudden onset of a serious illness or fever, or even concerns about the baby being lonely all appeared on the map of reasons for why families bedshare. "Peaceful," "comforting," "loving," and "protective" are words that showed up repeatedly in parental descriptions of what bedsharing means to them. "I work in an office all day long; cosleeping is a way to reconnect," said one mother.

Seeing the baby whenever you wake, watching the baby's chest rise up and down with each breath, hearing the baby (even if just a sigh or a faint sound), covering him if he's kicked off the blanket, wrapping your finger in his—these are the actions that sustain new parents and help them cherish the little life before them.

While many parents enjoy the closeness and bonding they are able to experience with their infant, the most prominent reason for cosleeping is that everyone gets more sleep.

Breastfeeding mothers and infants in particular get more rest when they cosleep, whether they are breastsleeping, using a cosleeping device, or simply have the crib in the same room with them. Think about it—it's much easier for mom to breastfeed bedside than to get up and walk down the hall to another room, and then try to resettle a baby who just wants to be touched by his or her mother.

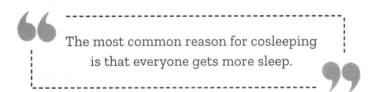

> The most common reason for cosleeping is that everyone gets more sleep.

Many mothers find it much easier to meet their breastfeeding goals while cosleeping, because they breastfeed more often and for longer periods of time in the first year of the infant's life than solitary-sleeping mothers.[105]

Epidemiological, laboratory, and observational studies reveal that, while babies certainly benefit from breastfeeding, mothers also experience short- and long-term health benefits from the act of breastfeeding.

# Breastfeeding is the Economical Way to Go

Breastfeeding saves at least $300 per month that otherwise would be spent on bottles, formula, or feeding costs, leading to enormous yearly family savings. It makes good financial sense, aside from all the health benefits for mother and infant alike.

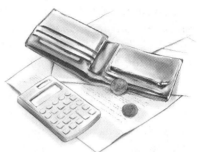

For example, breastfeeding helps return the mother's uterus to its pre-pregnancy size, works to help the mother retain iron, and delays the return of ovulation, which increases the birth interval. The shorter the intervals between feeds, the more powerful this contraceptive effect, called lactation amenorrhea, becomes.

Most importantly, breastfeeding helps to protect mothers from various kinds of reproductive cancers, especially breast cancer. The World Health Organization sponsored a study of 5,878 cases of breast cancer, comparing them with 8,216 controls (women who did not get cancer). They found that, as the number of lifetime months of breastfeeding increased, a woman's chances of getting breast cancer were diminished, especially if she breastfed for between 15–40 months of her life. If she did so, she had only a 30–40% chance of getting breast cancer compared with women who never breastfed, or who did so for only a few months.[147]

Another rather remarkable study describes a fishing village in Hong Kong where breastfeeding mothers do something we might think odd. They breastfeed their infants from only one breast. This amounts to the ultimate controlled experiment, since both breasts were exposed to the identical environmental factors and physiological experiences with only one exception: one breast was used for suckling and the other was not. Guess which breast did not become cancerous? Yes! The suckled breast seemed to be protected.[148]

A 2013 study by Dr. Melissa Bartick, Assistant Professor in Medicine at Harvard Medical School and Cambridge Health Alliance, found that suboptimal breastfeeding duration in the U.S. results in nearly 5,000 excess cases of breast cancer per year, and is also connected to nearly 14,000 excess heart attacks per year and over 50,000 cases of high blood pressure per year.[149]

Aside from the health benefits that come with more frequent breastfeeding, there are some reasons for breastsleeping that one might not think of, such as when the infants or parents are blind or deaf. One mother who participated in our study, sightless from birth, wrote: "How could I have ever mothered my darling baby without having him nestled up right near me? It gave me total fulfillment as a parent, and my son could not have cared less that I was sightless and, indeed, because of his utmost joy of me being close to him, I would often forget that I was, in fact, blind." The mother of a deaf and blind baby contributed: "I always felt a little weird about [my son] being in the dark and unable to hear, so once I gave up my 'preconceived notions' that children sleeping in their parents' bed was bad, bedtime has been much more peaceful."[36]

One mother of two deaf infants wrote: "I have two deaf boys, now five and eight. They both slept with us until this last year. We began [to breastsleep] by accident when nursing them made it much easier. When we found out the oldest was deaf we were so happy we had made that decision. Because they could not hear at night...they felt much more comfortable with us near them."

Peace of mind is significant, but the benefits for Mom and Dad don't stop there. Dr. Helen Ball's study of cosleeping fathers in England, the only study of its kind, found that the dads in her sample were initially reluctant to bedshare, yet they ended up finding the experience overall "more enjoyable than disruptive." She suggests that the intimate contact that dads can have with cosleeping babies helps them develop a strong social relationship with their infants that might otherwise be delayed during breastfeeding. Dr. Ball suggests that, "Triadic cosleeping arrangements may serve to ameliorate this effect [of a delayed relationship], and provide fathers who are motivated to do so the opportunity to experience intimate contact and prolonged close interaction with their newborn baby."[99]

# Part 4

How to Cosleep

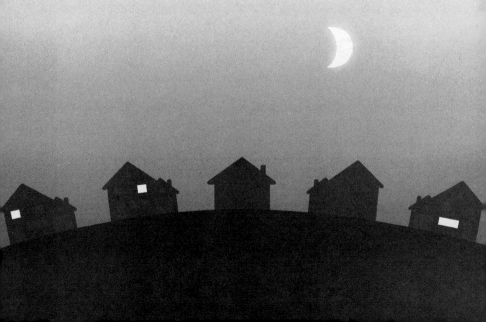

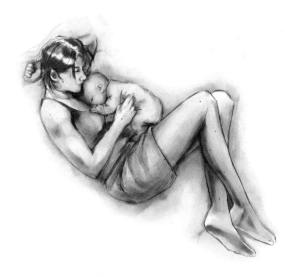

CHAPTER 8

# Safety First

## How to Breastsleep Safely

Keep in mind that every family naturally has its own set of goals, needs, and philosophies. Where a baby sleeps reflects the unique convergence of each family's values, the infant's feeding method, and multiple relational, psychological, and emotional characteristics of the parents and children. Even socioeconomic factors matter here, alongside, of course, the unique temperament and personality of the infant. This constellation of factors makes it impossible for even parents themselves to predict what type of sleeping arrangement will prove the most satisfying and beneficial for them.

Many parents discover that it is impractical to use a nursery, even if they have already invested a lot of time and money into preparing a beautiful space for their baby. Infants are biologically designed for physical contact. More than a pretty crib or bedroom, infants simply need their parents' proximity for their safety, development, and emotional security.

While I suggest that all parents keep their infants sleeping at least in the same room with them for at least the first six months, I don't feel that all families necessarily should or need to breastsleep. There are many other separate-surface cosleeping options to explore from which important benefits can still be gained. However, if you are the kind of parent who wants to feel the warmth, security, peace, and nurturing that comes with breastsleeping, then it is important to establish your bedsharing environment in a thoughtful, organized, and safe manner. By definition, breastsleeping occurs in an environment that is free from risk factors. In order to uphold the safety level of proper breastsleeping, you have to know what those risk factors are, and how to avoid them.

Let's start with the basics of creating a safe cosleeping environment. If you have a partner, having an honest talk about how each person feels about the sleeping arrangement is important. Also, keep in mind that decisions you make during pregnancy may not necessarily work out after the baby is born. Especially for first-time parents, experiencing the birth of your baby, holding your baby, and looking into his or her face can change everything you had decided.

If you transition into thinking you want to have your baby sleep in bed with you, I think it is appropriate for any adult who will share the bed to agree to take responsibility for the baby being there. Just like those little signs attached to cars that say "Baby on Board," before you enter the bed where a baby will sleep, be sure to think "Baby in Bed." Both parents need to share in responding to that baby's presence. It takes a conscious decision to be responsive, just as you decide not to roll out of your bed, or decide that you WILL wake up early before your plane leaves. Sleeping with a baby is more than a physical act, it is a mental act required of both parents in the bed, even though one may be responding to the baby more frequently than the other.

If you and your partner both agree to breastsleep, the first question must be: is your mattress firm enough? Dr. Ronald L. Somers, from Adelaide University in Australia, devised a clever way to find out, demonstrated in a video called "Babies and soft surfaces" posted on his YouTube channel. The process involves laying two full, one-liter milk or juice cartons on top of a stack of 12 CD disks, to test how far they sink into the mattress. If the computer disks sink to the point where the overhanging edge of the milk carton touches the mattress, that indicates that the bed is too soft and may be a suffocation hazard. Further details and a visual diagram can be found in Dr. Somers' 2012 publication in the *Australian and New Zealand Journal of Public Health*.[150]

Aside from the softness, another thing to look out for is the cleanliness of the mattress. For the sake of hygiene, it should be in good condition. It is also a good idea to check the label for potentially harmful materials.

Regardless of what mattress or sleeping arrangement you choose, always lay your baby on his or her back for sleep. It represents the species-wide natural sleep position for babies and helps facilitate breastfeeding, since a stomach-sleeping infant can't latch very easily, if at all, to the breast. Sleeping on their backs also induces babies to arouse more often, keeping them in a lighter-stage sleep and helping them awaken quickly following an apnea. Researchers have found that babies are at a much-reduced risk of succumbing to SIDS if they sleep on their backs, on a firm mattress with tight-fitting sheets, with their faces unobstructed by pillows, blankets, or stuffed animals, in a smoke-free setting.

If a mother smoked tobacco during her pregnancy, or smokes now, she should avoid bedsharing and instead have the baby sleep next to her on a separate surface. If the father smokes, it is likewise best to have the baby sleep alongside the bed, rather than in the bed. Dr. Peter Fleming's epidemiological study found that bedsharing with a smoking father also raises risk of SIDS to a problematic level.[151]

Smoking or ingesting marijuana may also pose a risk, although there is not enough research available to determine exactly how dangerous it is. According to a study in 2018, the main psychoactive ingredient in marijuana, THC, can remain in breastmilk for up to six days, and can accumulate in an infant's body fat. The authors speculate, "There is a concern for accumulation of the various cannabinoids in the nursing infant because of slow elimination from body fat stores and continuous daily exposure," but there have not been any studies confirming whether or not this THC build-up negatively affects brain development or contributes to SIDS in the same way as tobacco smoke.[152]

However, marijuana intake in any form, within a few hours

before bed, does increase the risk of SUID for bedsharing infants in the sense of altering a parent's awareness and ability to be sensitive to their baby's needs throughout the night. This is true for any drug.

Pathologist Dr. Claire Thornton made a statement about an infant who passed away in 2014 while bedsharing with her mother who had smoked marijuana before taking the infant to bed. Dr. Thornton said that, while the infant showed no signs of accidental or non-accidental injury or infection, and it was "impossible to tell" if the infant had been suffocated, the combination of marijuana and cosleeping created "an inestimably high risk" of SUID.[153]

Aside from the issue of smoking, if routinely breastsleeping, it is ideal to pull your bed into the center of the room—away from walls and surrounding furniture, strip away the metal or wood framework, and lay the box spring on the floor with the mattress on top. As shown by U.S. Consumer Product Safety Commission (CPSC) data, the most significant risk to a baby sleeping in a bed with an adult is not, as many assume, an adult overlaying or rolling onto the baby. Rather, the biggest risk is the baby becoming wedged or trapped between the mattress and a wall or a piece of furniture (like a bedside table), or the bed frame, headboard, or footboard.[154]

> The most significant risk to a baby sleeping in a bed with an adult is not, as many assume, an adult overlaying or rolling onto the baby.

If you are unable or unwilling to pull your bed apart and place it in the center of a room, at the very least check regularly for gaps and holes around your bed and inspect the furniture and other objects that surround your mattress. Make sure no furniture arrangement creates a gap between the furniture and the bed into which an infant could slip. Be sure that your headboard, footboard, and frame are tightly pressed to the mattress as well. Assume your baby will find a hole to fall into, if one exists.

Do not assume that pushing a mattress tightly against a wall is safe. Babies have suffocated when the parents did not notice the bed pulling away from the wall, leaving just enough space for the baby to become wedged in between.

When breastsleeping, it is also important to remember to set the thermostat a bit lower. Your own body next to the baby's acts to keep the baby warm; excessive warmth for an infant increases the chances of SIDS. Light blankets are best, and little sleep suits might work well for your baby as long as the infant's arms are not constricted. Infants should always be able to swipe at objects obstructing their nose or mouth. Keep your baby away from duvets or heavy blankets that can flop over and cover his or her face, and use hard, angular pillows pushed well above the infant's head. Also, be sure to keep other children and pets out of your bed when your baby is sleeping in it.

If you have extremely long hair, you should tie it up in a way that does not dangle like a cord near the infant. I know of one occasion where a baby got so tangled up in the mother's long hair that the father had to cut her hair off to save the infant from being

## The Consequences of Unsafe Bedsharing

**DO NOT BEDSHARE, even in the form of breastsleeping, if there is any space between the bed and the wall or other furniture where the baby could roll and become trapped**.

Make sure the mattress fits tightly against the headboard and the footboard, and remove the bed frame if at all possible.

If you do not take proper precautions,
the following could happen to your baby:

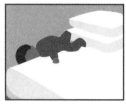
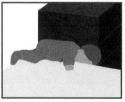
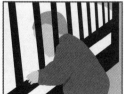

*Entrapment between bed and wall*

*Entrapment between bed and object*

*Entrapment in footboard of bed*

strangled. The baby was resuscitated, but it was a very close call.

Careful considerations also need to be made if either adult sleeping in the bed is obese. Excess weight might create a depression or space that the baby may roll into while sleeping. A particularly stiff mattress may compensate for this situation. No hard and fast rule about parental obesity and bedsharing can be empirically justified, except where no breastfeeding occurs or other risk factors exist or predominate, in which case bedsharing should be avoided. These families can cosleep by placing the baby on a surface near the bed rather than in the bed itself. One study of the relationship between obesity and cosleeping on a couch (a dangerous cosleeping environment for anyone) shows a tremendously elevated risk if both factors are present, although the data also documents multiple other independent risk factors.[155]

If you or your partner feel cramped in your bed, or if the bed is smaller than a queen size, then it is best not to bedshare. You should have enough room to spread apart. The new folded mattresses or quilted mattresses appear not to be flat or stable enough for maximum protection of your baby, so it is best to avoid sleeping with your baby on those particular mattresses. Never bedshare, even in the form of breastsleeping, if you sleep on a waterbed. I hope someday authorities and manufacturers will begin to think about bed furniture that is, by design, safer for babies.

For information about naptime safety, see Chapter 11.

# The Proper Way to Bedshare

*An idealized sketch of bedsharing shows parents who do not smoke, are sober, have chosen to bedshare, and are breastfeeding their baby. The bed frame has been completely removed and the mattress has been placed at the center of the room away from walls and furniture. Light blankets and firm, square pillows are being used. No older children, pets, or stuffed animals are in the bed.*

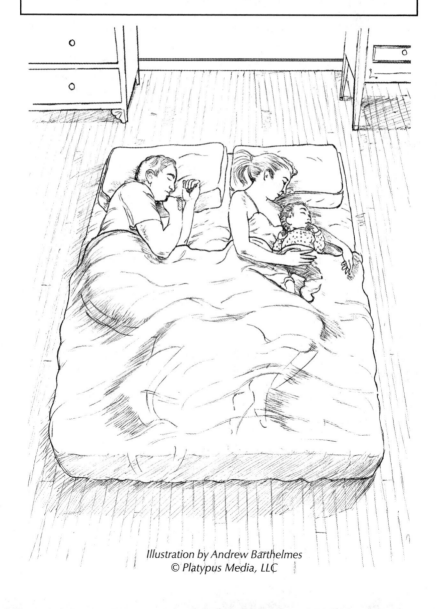

*Illustration by Andrew Barthelmes*
*© Platypus Media, LLC*

# Breastsleeping Dos and Don'ts

## DO:

 Ask your partner or anyone else sharing the bed if they are comfortable with the baby sleeping there, and if they are willing to share responsibility for the baby's safety throughout the night.

 Make sure your baby is sleeping on a clean, firm, non-quilted surface, with plenty of space for all occupants. A mattress in the middle of the room with no frame is ideal.

 Tie up long hair in a bun or other style that will not be able to wrap around the infant. For extremely long hair, even a ponytail or braid may pose a hazard.

 Thoroughly check for any gaps or bars that may cause entrapment.

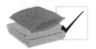 Remove stuffed animals or dolls, heavy blankets, thick duvets, extra pillows, or any other objects that may pose a suffocation risk. Light sheets and breathable blankets are acceptable.

 Keep pets out of the bedroom if they are able to climb onto the bed.

 Provide a smoke-free environment for your baby. If anyone sharing the bed smokes tobacco (no matter where or when they smoke), have your baby sleep on a separate surface.

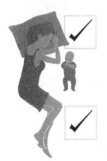 Place your baby on his or her back to sleep. Position the baby's head by the breastsleeping mother's chest, and not by the pillows. When breastfeeding in bed, make sure the baby returns to this position at the end of each feed.

Place your baby between the breastsleeping mother and the edge of the bed, so the baby is not between two individuals. If the second adult is fully and enthusiastically invested in the baby being there, and is confident that they can respond to the infant's needs, this may be more flexible.

 Assess your ability to respond to your baby throughout the night.

# DON'T:

Do not breastsleep if you or your partner smoke, or if you smoked tobacco during your pregnancy.

Do not breastsleep if anyone sharing the bed has consumed sedatives, medications, alcohol, marijuana, or any substance that causes altered consciousness or marked drowsiness.

Do not breastsleep if anyone sharing the bed, especially the breastsleeping mother, is ill or tired to the point where it would be difficult to respond to the baby.

Don't leave any space between the bed and the wall where the baby could roll and become trapped. Make sure that the mattress fits tightly against the headboard and footboard, and remove the bed frame if at all possible.

Do not breastsleep if a parent is markedly obese, unless he or she feels confident that the mattress is stiff enough to compensate for the greater weight differential.

Do not allow older siblings who do not understand the risks of suffocation to sleep in the same bed with infants less than one year old.

Do not breastsleep if pets are able or likely to climb into the bed.

Don't use thick bedding, and don't allow anything to cover the head or face of the baby. Sheets and blankets should be porous, preferably cotton. In cold weather, use layers of thin bedding rather than one heavier blanket.

Don't dress your baby too warmly or set the thermostat too high. If you are comfortable, your baby probably is too. Remember, close bodily contact increases body temperature.

Never leave long hair down or wear nightclothes with strings or ties. These pose a strangulation risk for the baby.

Never place babies alone in an adult bed. Babies should always sleep under supervision.

———— ❯ ————

# Is There a Risk of Rolling Onto My Baby?

To claim that there is no chance of an adult ever overlaying (rolling onto) a baby, even in an otherwise safe set of circumstances, would be untrue. However, it would be similarly untrue to claim that an infant could never accidentally be killed while traveling in an automobile, or could never die from other common, socially-acceptable activities. In each case, the dangers are specific, known, and can mostly be avoided. In the case of automobile travel, strapping infants correctly into a consumer safety-approved car seat and not driving while under the influence makes car transportation worth the relatively small risk such travel imposes.

We know that sleeping with a baby on a couch, sofa, recliner, chair, or waterbed is always dangerous, and that any sleeping arrangement involving an infant can be made dangerous. However, many are not inherently so.

A mother does not, by default, pose a risk to her baby, whether sleeping on the same surface or alongside her baby on a separate surface. As we know from research by Dr. Valdes-Dapena[91] and experiments by Dr. Rosenblith and Dr. Anderson-Huntington,[90] (see Chapter 6) a committed, sober caregiver can easily notice and respond to an infant's distress in a dangerous situation. Our own NICHD-funded studies show that breastsleeping mothers are able to sense, detect, and respond to the proximity of their babies, even in the deepest stages of sleep. I would argue that a sober, informed, dedicated mother—especially one who is breastfeeding—is value added in a cosleeping arrangement, and not an inherent risk as has been portrayed by medical authorities. Anyone who thinks a mother lying next to her infant is always an unacceptable risk has been misled to believe that breastsleeping is a pathology, or abnormal behavior, when, in fact, it is a fundamental human adaptation that should be the default arrangement.

Anthropological evidence, comprised of cross-cultural, cross-species, and evolutionary data, suggests that mothers and infants are designed to respond to each other's presence. This is a biological fact, empirically demonstrable. It is evidenced in reports by mothers themselves, describing how their attentiveness and interventions while bedsharing potentially saved their infant's life[36] (see Appendix IV). It is true that bedsharing is less stable and requires careful preparation, but that does not necessarily make it unsafe. I like to remind people that if same-surface cosleeping were too dangerous, infants and parents would have evolved some biologically-based alternative or humankind would have gone extinct. As it is, infant-parent cosleeping in all of its diverse forms continues to be the globally preferred sleeping arrangement for human and other mammal mother-baby pairs.

> If same-surface cosleeping were too dangerous, infants and parents would have evolved some biologically-based alternative or humankind would have gone extinct.

In well-documented, worldwide cultural records and recorded information about nonhuman primates, I have never been able to find a word or phrase suggesting an occurrence of Sudden Infant Death Syndrome before the development of industrialized societies. I have also never found any reports from more simply-organized societies—such as contemporary hunters and gatherers—that describe a mother accidentally suffocating her baby by cosleeping. It is hard to believe that it has never happened at all in these societies, as even a rare occurrence would seem likely, but SIDS and infant suffocation seem to be phenomena mainly familiar to those of us living in Western industrialized nations. These phenomena are particularly prevalent in cultural sub-groups that are structurally and historically marginalized or impoverished due to racism and inter-generational trauma.

Where breastsleeping finds expression in less industrial contexts, the practice continues to provide life-saving nutritional, immunological, neuro-developmental, and physiological advantages. We can still bedshare and achieve these benefits in our industrialized societies but, for us, taking precautions and staying informed is much more important. Breastsleeping evolved to be the predominant and most adaptive human sleeping and feeding arrangement, but modern furniture and sleep accouterments, drug and alcohol use, formula and bottle-feeding, and smoking were not part of the equation during most of human evolution. We must take these factors into consideration when talking about overlaying risk and when determining what a safe breastsleeping environment looks like in an urban, Western, industrialized setting.

Modern societies and sleeping environments and the social and physical conditions within which bedsharing occurs—especially among the urban poor—forces professionals to be very guarded when discussing bedsharing or cosleeping. Given that I do not know the specific conditions and circumstances in which every family lives, I make sure I do not directly recommend that any particular parent bedshare. It is one thing, however, to explicitly talk about when it is not safe to bedshare, and a very different thing to try to expunge such an important behavioral experience altogether, claiming that it is inevitably dangerous.

I have argued throughout my career that health professionals do not have the right—nor the evidence—to sweep all forms of bedsharing into the same taxonomic bin. Time and time again there are explanations of infant deaths that require reference to the presence of multiple dangerous risk factors.[58] I stress that a distinction must be made between the inherently protective and beneficial nature of the mother-infant cosleeping relationship and the conditions in which it occurs, which can range from extremely safe to extremely dangerous and risky. For example, the condition of the sleeping surface, the frame of mind of the adult cosleepers, and the family's reasons for cosleeping are all very important in assessing the relative safety of a bedsharing arrangement.

As mentioned in an earlier chapter, many of the ongoing disagreements regarding bedsharing stem from the mixed results of epidemiological case control studies. These studies significantly undercount the number of infants who bedshared and survived without incident. They are also not easily comparable, containing enormous variation in the cultural context, definitions of variables, questions included, and presence of extraneous risk factors.

There are many situations within which bedsharing poses too many risks, but studies that include relevant details of the circumstances within which infants die—such as specific details on infant sleep location or parental alcohol, tobacco, or drug use—have shown only slightly elevated or no difference in risk for bedsharing infants of breastfeeding, non-smoking, sober mothers.[156]

In 2013, one of the biggest names in SIDS research, Dr. Abraham Bergman, wrote an editorial in response to an article by Dr. Eve Colson, both published in the *Journal of the American Medical Association* (JAMA).[67] Dr. Colson's research team reported that from 1993 through 2010, the overall trend of U.S. caregivers sharing a bed with their infants had significantly increased. Because of their belief that bedsharing increases infant mortality, the authors called for increased efforts by pediatricians to discourage the practice. Dr. Bergman found the report "disquieting." In his editorial, he wrote: "the evidence linking bedsharing per se to the increased risk for infant death is shaky, and certainly insufficient to condemn a widespread cultural practice that has its own benefits."[157] Dr. Colson's paper, which was primarily focused on increased rates of bedsharing, without any direct evidence about the safety of the practice, pushed well beyond what could be said about risk from the data the authors actually provided. It turned out to be a polemic against bedsharing, rather than drawing inferences as to why parents might be disregarding the AAP's warnings against the practice. Dr. Bergman went on to write, "...it is becoming clear to many doctors and researchers that non-uniform and unverifiable information on the causes of death... led to conclusions about bedsharing that are not supported."

While there is evidence that accidental suffocation from overlaying can and does occur in bedsharing situations, in the overwhelming number of cases there are also extremely unsafe sleeping conditions present. This includes situations where adults were not aware that the infant was in the bed, were drunk or desensitized by drugs, or were indifferent to the baby's presence. And, of course, suffocation is more likely if the parent and infant sleep on a sofa or couch together, which is no doubt the deadliest form of cosleeping.

This is why it is important to establish your cosleeping environment in a safe and organized manner (see "Breastsleeping Dos and Don'ts"). If another adult is in the bed, the second adult should be made aware of the presence of the baby, and it should never be assumed that the other adult knows the baby is present.

Toddlers or pets should not be permitted to sleep in the parental bed with an infant, as they are unaware of the dangers of suffocation and pose a risk of overlaying. It would be perhaps even more dangerous for an infant and a toddler to sleep alone together in the same bed.

Finally, it is not a pleasant thought to consider, but I always think that it is important to consider how you would react if, by chance, an infant died from SIDS while sleeping next to you. Would you assume that you suffocated the infant? Or would you know that you did not, that the infant died independently of your presence? If you are disinclined to believe that SIDS could occur in the bedsharing context, just as it can occur under perfectly safe solitary-sleeping conditions, then perhaps it might be best to have your infant cosleep next to you on a separate surface rather than in your bed. Regardless of what you decide, it is important to think about the possibility, no matter how remote and unlikely such a scenario may be. SIDS can indeed occur where safe bedsharing, breastfeeding, and optimal care for the infant take place, making this a question worth discussing with your partner.

There is no infant sleep environment that is completely risk free, even when all known unsafe factors are removed. However, the right to consider what risk factors are present, and to weigh those risks in relationship to individual bedsharing circumstances, belongs with the parent—not with external authorities. Guidance from professionals researching these issues may be appropriate, but dictatorial negative warnings or insults are not helpful. It is not okay for civil or medical authorities to speak as if parents are incapable of creating a safe sleep space or of using scientific information to weigh the potential risks and benefits of bedsharing in the context of their own family.

Let me end on a positive note: breastsleeping among non-smoking mothers, specifically for the purpose of breastfeeding, with all else being safe, is the ideal form of bedsharing. Both mother and baby can benefit, with the baby getting more of mother's precious milk, and both mother and baby getting more sleep.

# Choosing Your Cosleeping Arrangement

*Follow the flowchart to discover whether you should bedshare or whether you should explore separate-surface cosleeping options. Remember, YOU are the best judge of what sleeping arrangement will work for your infant. This chart merely shows you how to minimize risk according to current research and encourages you to think about risks and potential benefits in your own specific circumstances.*

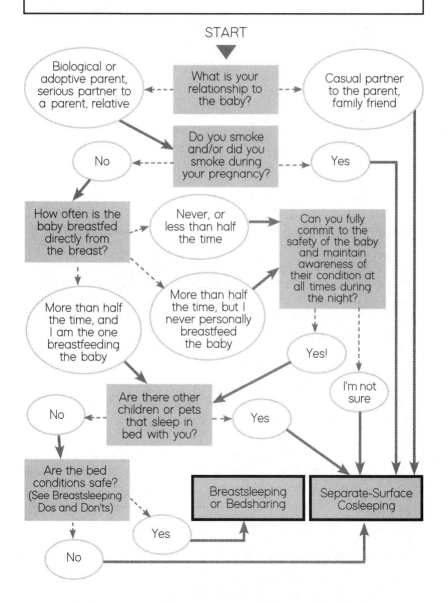

# For Those of You Who Choose to Breastsleep

If, at this point, you have made the decision to breastsleep, there are a few things I want to reiterate. The first of these is that there are more risk factors involved in bedsharing than there are in separate-surface cosleeping situations. Unlike a crib environment that is designed for one small body, bedsharing is less socially and structurally stable. Risk factors must be identified and assessed by parents if they decide they want to share a bed with their baby.

> There are more risk factors involved in bedsharing than there are in separate-surface cosleeping situations.

Cosleeping is generally talked about in the context of the home, but even in the hospital, risks must be taken into account. Aside from the mother being exhausted, and perhaps still a bit anaesthetized from the drugs used during labor, hospital beds are generally unsafe for infants. The narrowness and height of the bed, along with the lack of cosleeping safety measures, make it problematic for mothers to drift in and out of sleep at this time.

While it remains critical for mothers to have immediate, sustained contact with their infants in order to optimize their breastmilk production, the beginnings of attachment, and milk let-down, falling asleep with an infant can quickly become a liability issue for hospitals.

Once you return home, where you have more control over the sleep environment, it is crucial to your child's safety that you can anticipate possible threats. For example, if you choose to breastsleep for any time during the night, how likely is it that a sibling or another adult will be in or enter the bed? In such cases, these other bed-sharers might not be as diligent as you are, or they might not have the capacity to protect the infant during sleep. Similarly, how likely is it that a family pet will jump on the bed, causing a rearrangement of blankets, pillows, or bodies that inadvertently pushes the baby into harm's way? By assessing these risks, you can lessen the chance that your child will be in danger. You can eliminate risk factors (for example, closing the door to your room so the family pet can't enter, or crating the pet within the room), but if these risks can't be avoided in your bed, you can place your baby on a separate sleep surface like a crib or bassinet alongside the bed.

I cannot emphasize enough that most infant deaths in the U.S. that occurred in adult beds happened due to the infant being wedged between the mattress and a headboard or footboard, wall, or nightstand. If breastsleeping is to be a routine, and if all other risk factors are eliminated, then the adult bed is best placed in the middle of the room, away from all walls or furniture. The mattress should be out of its frame and should be covered with simple, lightweight blankets, tight-fitting sheets, and firm pillows.

Please remember, if you smoked tobacco during or after pregnancy, if you or your partner take any kind of drugs or alcohol before bed, or if your baby is not breastfed, then separate-surface cosleeping is the safest form of cosleeping for your family.

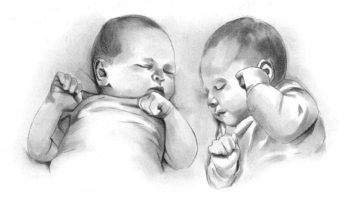

## CHAPTER 9

# Special Considerations

## Breastsleeping With Twins or Multiples

As with any aspect of caring for twins or multiples, there are added challenges to breastsleeping. My general recommendations are to place at least one multiple back in the crib or bassinet after feeding, sleeping with one multiple at a time; to place both or all infants back in the same crib or bassinet to cobed with each other (see the next section); or to place two or more bassinets next to each other.

If regularly breastsleeping with your twins or multiples, it is essential to have a king-size bed and a partner who is more than a passive participant, who has agreed to work with you to take responsibility for knowing exactly where each baby is at all times.

If the second adult does not agree to actively participate in taking care of at least one multiple, but you want to continue to breastsleep, then do not leave one infant between yourself and your partner. Have all multiples in front of you so that you can curve your body around them and shield them from your bed-mate.

Keeping your infants at some distance from each other will

be important too, only because it is likely for one baby to want to snuggle close to you, and, in the process, snuggle perhaps too close to his or her sibling. Use only the lightest of blankets to ensure free air passage for all infants. The fact that hungry infants are quite capable of mistaking a sibling's nose for a breast is worth preparing for, because, as strange or as funny as it may seem, one twin sucking on the nose of the other can quickly dehydrate the other.

I recommend that if there is a partner in the bed who has no interest in monitoring or taking responsibility for any multiples, after each breastfeed (and if not breastfeeding at all), it is best to place the infants back in a bassinet or crib to cobed. Lactation consultant Karen Gromada has written a wonderful book on parenting multiples if you are interested in more information.[158]

## Cobedding Twins

From a scientific point of view, this is an area that is rarely investigated. The term for cosleeping twins is *cobedding*. It occurs when two bodies of equal size and weight share the same crib. How cobedding functions, and its role in infant development and safety, is very different from other forms of cosleeping that have been discussed through the majority of this book.

Twins and multiples generally are, for reasons still unknown, associated with a higher risk for SIDS. This makes questions about which sleep environment might best protect them, and which will put them at increased risk, especially critical. Questions pertaining to cobedding often emerge in conversations about premature births, as many twins are also born premature. Prematurity is the leading cause of hospitalization during the neonatal period, and is responsible for up to 75% of neonatal illnesses and deaths, so this is an area in need of much further exploration.[159]

The challenge of all newborns making their way from the womb to the worldly environment is to re-establish some kind of "biorhythmic balance" by stabilizing the functions of sleep-wake cycles, eating patterns, blood chemistry levels, and respiratory and heart rates. Two teams of researchers have argued that the mutual sensory exchanges that are facilitated by cobedding may enhance the ability of any one twin to accomplish this task. The researchers found that, similar to what is observed to occur in the womb, cobedded twins move close together, touch and suck on each other, hold each other, and hug one another. These actions improve breathing, help infants use energy more efficiently, and

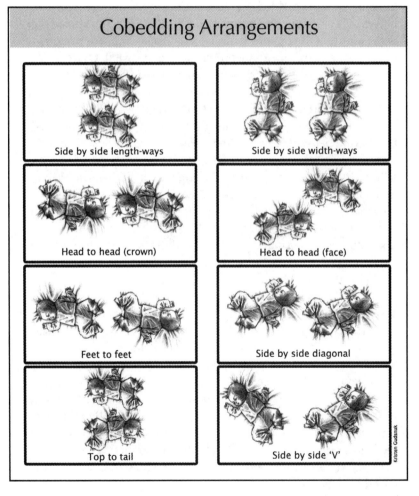

*Fig. 4.1 Drawing by Kristen Gudsnuk, modeled after Ball, H.L. (2006), "Caring for twin infants: sleeping arrangements and their implications." Evidence-Based Midwifery 4(1),10-16. Courtesy of: Evidence-Based Midwifery.*

generally reduce the twins' stress levels. This is valuable because stress can negatively impact growth and development; increased cortisol production alters thermal regulation, sleep duration, breathing, and heart rate in negative ways.

Studies done by Dr. Helen Ball show that twins smile at each other and are often awake at the same time, supporting several anecdotal reports by parents of twins that their own infants prefer to be together and that their babies settle better and sleep more soundly when cobedded. Given the challenges of caring for two babies, as Dr. Ball points out from her studies, it is not surprising that parents will come to practice any behavioral care pattern which tends to maximize their own sleep and ease the burden of caring for and feeding two babies simultaneously.[160, 161, 162]

Nowadays, recommendations against cobedding often illustrate cultural biases against cosleeping in general. Medical authorities assume—without any data—that if some instances of bedsharing between an adult and a baby are dangerous, then two infants of equal body size must likewise pose a mutual threat. When there is a gap in our knowledge, or little information is available, medical and non-medical recommendations quickly rely on generalizations, stereotypes, and anecdotal information, which is then passed on as if proven to be scientifically true. In this case, studies of bedsharing involving adults and infants are being applied to the question of whether or not it is safe or beneficial for twins to share a crib.

Some hospital nursery wards are already assuming that the AAP's recommendation against bedsharing applies to twins. In fact, no twin studies were considered as the basis for those guidelines, and no evidence-based considerations have thus far been used to justify hospital policies that argue against cobedding.

To my knowledge, Dr. Helen Ball is one of very few researchers who have detailed empirical data on cobedding twins, including fundamental physiological data comparing cobedded infants with separate-sleeping twins. The cobedding sketches in this section are based on her original work. I highly recommend that you read her two studies carefully before you decide how or if you want to cobed your twins.[160, 161, 162]

## Cosleeping With an Adopted Baby

Depending on their ages and experiences, adopted infants and children may have heightened needs for affection and contact; however, if they are older, they may not be used to intimacy. Watch carefully how your child reacts to you and respond accordingly. It is also helpful, where possible, to know your child's history and assess what special needs or processes may be required to integrate the child into your family and to establish secure, safe, and trustworthy new relationships.

If you have adopted an infant and not a child, of course, there is no difference. Regardless of cultural origin, place of birth, or ethnicity, all babies have the same needs. Since attachment between any of us can be greatly enhanced by contact, cosleeping behavior can greatly facilitate the developing bond between your adopted baby and yourself. Bedsharing without breastfeeding for an adopted infant should be avoided, but using cosleeping devices or otherwise roomsharing may be a safe, fulfilling option.

It may be the case that adoption agencies require infants or children to have their own rooms. But you will be joining millions of parents whose nighttime care and associations with their children are hardly defined nor limited by the number of bedrooms they have, or where a crib may be located.

## Cosleeping With Premature or Underweight Babies

In almost all of the epidemiological studies that I am aware of, infants who are premature or small for their gestational age constitute a disproportionate number of SIDS victims and victims of SUID in bedsharing situations. The reasons for this are not yet known, and could possibly include in-utero developmental events or assaults to the fetal nervous system, some of which are induced by maternal smoking.

Routine breastsleeping does not seem to contribute to the survival of these more fragile infants, so it is best avoided. Place your premature or underweight baby right next to your bed on a different surface, but not in bed with you. Skin-to-skin contact while awake, however, is extremely protective, and sensory exchanges with an adult are known to be clinically beneficial

# What Can I Do to Make Bedtime Easier for My Premature Baby?

It is not safe to have a very small, fragile, premature baby sleeping next to an adult in a Western bed. The strategy I recommend to keep them safe and close is to have them sleep alongside the bed in a cosleeping device (see Appendix II). Some cosleeping devices, like the Arm's Reach® Cosleeper® Bassinet,* have the added advantage of providing space to keep medical equipment and other items needed for preemie care.

The infant-parent sensory exchanges and monitoring by the parent that occurs during separate-surface cosleeping, coupled with breastfeeding and episodes of sustained skin-to-skin contact while awake, are about as good as it gets for your premature infant. When awake, you and your partner should hold and be in contact with your baby as much as possible. Contact isn't just nice, it is a positive factor in the regulation of your baby's immature physiology. It is also the closest sensory experience the infant can get to being back in the mother's womb, from which he or she was prematurely evicted.

*I need to disclose here that I have been a paid consultant regarding the safety aspects of the Arm's Reach® Cosleeper® for many years now. I mention this brand because it is the only such infant sleep structure for which I personally know the safety record. This particular crib, which attaches to the parental bed, has an unblemished safety record insofar as no infant deaths or injuries have ever been reported during the near 30 years it has been on the market— an amazing feat, indeed.

to developmentally disadvantaged infants. The more holding, carrying, and breastmilk made available for these special babies, and the more physical interactions you have with them, the better. In multiple studies, premature babies receiving skin-to-skin contact while the caregiver was awake reduced infant mortality by a whopping 36%.[122] These results are consistent with Dr. Tiffany Field's classic study of the effects of daily 15-minute massages on full term infants. In her study, which has been replicated several times, massaged infants experienced 47% more average daily weight gain than non-massaged infants. It is nothing less than amazing just how much enhanced holding, carrying, and touching can do to promote good health among human infants, as I have emphasized throughout this book.

# Part 5

## Fitting Cosleeping Into Your Life

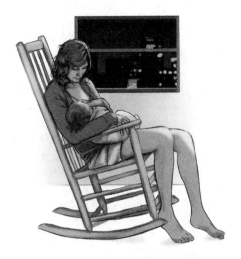

CHAPTER 10

# Infant Sleep, Nighttime Care Practices, and Cultural Context

When it comes to their infant's sleep, parents living in Western industrialized societies (particularly in the U.S.) may well be the most obsessed, the most well-read, the most educated, the most judgmental, the most exhausted, and the most disappointed on the planet! The absurdity of our obsession becomes apparent in the book, *Babyhood*, written by Paul Reiser (star of the old series *Mad About You*). If I could, I would give Reiser an Academy Award for providing the funniest and most entertaining analysis of this modern parenting struggle. He says:

> "Getting your child to sleep becomes such a blinding obsession, I myself would often lose sight of the bigger picture: What is the actual goal here? Constant sleep? No awake time? Zero consciousness? I mean, we must accept that at some point babies have to be awake. They didn't come to the planet just to sleep.

"Are we determined to get them asleep just so we can get a taste of what life was like before we had kids? Because if we are, then tell me again—why did we have a kid? Just to lie there and look soft and fuzzy? We could have just gotten, say, a peach. A St. Bernard. A narcoleptic houseguest. Or why not just get a huge chenille bathrobe? Chenille bathrobes are fuzzy and just lie there—why don't we just get us one of those and name it Michael?"

The true irony is that the usual recommendations for getting your infant or child to sleep promote parenting approaches that actually perpetuate the problems sleep clinicians are asked to solve.

Earlier in the book I made the point that, due to the convergence of a variety of cultural, social, religious, economic, and historical factors unique to the Western world, the nighttime infant care practices recommended by medical professionals became one and the same with the social values and ideologies of the culture that produced them.[8, 98, 115, 116] By the early 20th Century, the general opinion was that infants should be taught right from the beginning to sleep through the night, to be on a routine, and to expect few—if any—nighttime interventions from parents. For example, a common, relatively recent recommendation has been to *never let an infant fall asleep at the breast,* which directly conflicts with the practice of breastsleeping. It offers no proven benefits for infants and clearly reflects a long history of infant care recommendations based on social ideology, personal preference, and folk myth. I honestly can't imagine why anyone would make such a suggestion, forcing parents to deny themselves and their infants an evolved human behavior.

Similarly, almost century-old Western baby manuals somehow continue to influence modern ideas about infant sleep. In 1935, Marianna Wheeler wrote in her book *The Baby, His Care and Training,* "The constant handling of an infant is not good for him. The less he is lifted, held and passed from one pair of hands to another, the better, as while he is so young his bones are soft, and constant handling does not tend to improve their development nor the shapeliness of his little body. The newborn infant should spend the greater portion of his life on the bed." From the same decade, the anonymous author of *The Motherhood*

*Book,* published in London, stated: "Babies should be trained from their earliest days to sleep regularly and should never be woken in the night for feeding....And baby should be given his own bedroom from the very beginning. He should never be brought into the living room at night."

In the classic *Baby and Child Care* book, originally published in 1946, Dr. Benjaman Spock said this to millions of mothers: "You know more than you think you do....Don't be afraid to trust your own common sense. Bringing up your child won't be a complicated job if you take it easy, trust your own instincts, and follow the directions your doctor gives you!" This pervasive message, seemingly intended to give mothers confidence, actually creates more uncertainty when a parent's instincts don't match the doctor's orders.

Past recommendations from health professionals and parenting experts were, of course, predicated and made possible by the assumption that bottle-feeding baby formula or cow's milk would be the preferred, if not superior, feeding method—and, during the last century, it was indeed preferred.

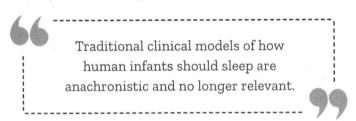

Traditional clinical models of how human infants should sleep are anachronistic and no longer relevant.

Yet, today, the situation is very different, with about 81% of American mothers leaving the hospital breastfeeding. This figure is higher in many other Western industrialized societies. Even without considering that at some point in the first three months of life most infants are likely to navigate their way into their mothers' beds, breastfed infants exhibit vastly different sleep patterns than infants who are fed artificial milk. Therefore, traditional clinical models of how human infants should sleep are anachronistic and no longer relevant.

The image and assumption of the bottle-fed, solitary-sleeping baby—illustrated by the ever-present *sleep like a baby* mantra— is a tenacious cultural icon, with many careers staked on its validity. Nevertheless, it has become clear with the re-emergence of breastfeeding that this cultural image represents an infant disarticulated from the only environment (sleep- and feeding-wise) to which he or she is adapted: the mother's body. It is what author Richard Dawkins calls a cultural meme—not a viral internet joke, as the term has come to mean, but an innovation or a novel idea that gets transmitted across generations, with or without any empirical evidence.[163] Unfortunately, this meme continues to prevail in various professional and popular manifestations of normal human infant sleep, leaving parents to essentially fend for themselves in finding answers for why their infants, especially when breastfed, often refuse to sleep alone or through the night.

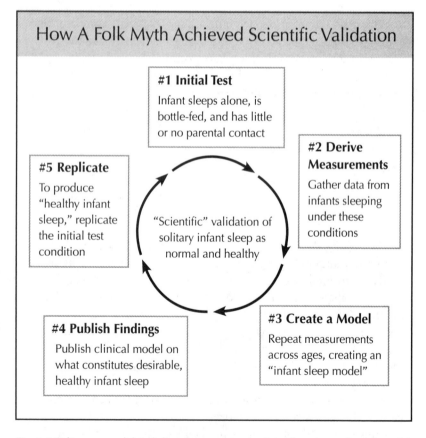

## How A Folk Myth Achieved Scientific Validation

**#1 Initial Test**
Infant sleeps alone, is bottle-fed, and has little or no parental contact

**#2 Derive Measurements**
Gather data from infants sleeping under these conditions

**#3 Create a Model**
Repeat measurements across ages, creating an "infant sleep model"

**#4 Publish Findings**
Publish clinical model on what constitutes desirable, healthy infant sleep

**#5 Replicate**
To produce "healthy infant sleep," replicate the initial test condition

"Scientific" validation of solitary infant sleep as normal and healthy

*Fig. 5.1 Solitary, consolidated sleep became standardized based on a flawed model of what healthy infant sleep looks like—one that ignored infants' biological needs.*

❨

# The Social Construct of Sleeping Through the Night

Not even half of all babies actually sleep through the night, at least not in the first year of life. One of the most careful and best-designed recent studies on the issue of when human infants sleep through the night was published in *Pediatrics* in 2018.[164] Their aim was to investigate the proportion of infants who slept in six- to eight-hour sleep blocks at 6 and 12 months of age. The research team also looked at these sleeping patterns in relation to mental and psychomotor development, maternal mood, and breastfeeding. They found that 27% to 57% of 6- and 12-month-old infants did not sleep through the night. They also found no association between sleeping through the night and mental development, psychomotor development, or maternal mood. And, importantly, for clarifying the relationship between breastfeeding and sleep behavior, they found that sleeping through the night was associated with a lower rate of breastfeeding.

The authors concluded that as a "potential protective strategy" to eliminate maternal worries associated with infants who will not sleep through the night, all mothers should be told (as my own book has argued) that the normal development of the sleep-wake cycle occurs late in the first year of life for most infants. Hence, parents need not focus on sleep training methods and other interventions, because failing to sleep through the night is actually more appropriate. The authors put it this way: "The transition to parenthood is a vulnerable period of life and it could be reassuring for parents to learn that in a typically developing cohort up to 36.6% of infants do not sleep six consecutive hours at six months, and up to 29.7% do not at the age of 12 months." While this will need to be replicated before it substantially proves anything, this team has certainly illuminated important evidence about normative human infant biology.

While night waking is not a sign of a clinical problem that requires professional treatment, it is still interesting to ask, what does cause infants to wake at night? If infants wake up easily, and this is always a relative description, then it is likely biologically appropriate and influenced by feeding method (bottle, breast, or mixed) and general comfort level (diaper condition and/or hunger). A variety of scientific studies indicate that the baby's own internal needs—to feed, to find reassurance, or to breathe— are as much influencing factors in night waking as sleep location.

Recall that breastfed infants wake up much more frequently and at shorter intervals than bottle-fed infants. Cow's milk is designed for a cow's brain growth and body growth rates. It has the wrong concentrations of proteins and micro and macro nutrients, as well as maternal, home-grown antibodies, and other immune factors that protect against the specific microbes from which the human baby needs defense. The kinds of proteins in each milk also have different molecular structures, so, in addition to being mismatched with the infant's biology, babies cannot digest cow's milk as easily as breastmilk. Cow's milk takes longer for the infant to process, leading to larger intervals between feedings. Breastmilk, however, provides just the right composition for that growing infant brain, which doubles in size in the first year.

Barring the presence of more serious neurological problems, eventually all children will sleep through the night and adjust themselves to their family's sleep schedule. No child needs to be sleep trained, or put through a controlled crying or controlled comforting training course, though I realize some professionals claim that the sooner a baby learns to "self soothe," the better for the child's healthy development. As I pointed out earlier, this idea actually leads to suboptimal breastfeeding and conflicts with AAP recommendations that an infant, if possible, breastfeeds for a full year. Obviously, many circumstances, including access to resources, will make this possible or not, but we should avoid adding additional barriers to this goal—especially when there is no evidence that sleeping through the night has any effect on mental or psychomotor development.

A professional might even say that, at four to six months, a child should be sleeping through the night alone, but as we know this is a slightly different version of the same cultural meme— a personal opinion with no validity other than what it might mean to the person saying it. Sleeping through the night may be convenient for parents, so they may choose to practice any number of sleep training methods to speed up the natural process of sleep consolidation. But I can assure you that it has no positive benefits for the child, that are not also obtained through a child's own natural social and biological development.

In my mind, the stress that infants experience during sleep training, which is reflected in higher cortisol levels, makes such interventions not worth the result. Psychology professor Dr. Wendy Middlemiss and colleagues monitored 25 mothers and their infants as they began a sleep training program. During the first three days, both mothers and infants experienced significantly raised cortisol levels. But an interesting difference between infants and their mothers occurred on, or close to, day three.

On the surface, the infants stopped protesting the isolation (i.e., stopped crying). While the mothers' cortisol levels dropped upon seeing that their babies appeared to be content, analysis of the infants' saliva told a very different story: the infants' cortisol levels remained as high as before. In other words, while it looked like all was well for the infants, the amount of cortisol in their saliva was significantly high. What the infants showed on the surface wasn't what they were actually feeling.[165]

On top of this, research findings describing the normalcy of frequent awakenings make putting a young child through a cruel experience like sleep training totally unnecessary, especially considering that it has a better chance of failing than succeeding, and a high likelihood of creating unintended problems.

> No child needs to be sleep trained or put through a controlled crying or controlled comforting training course.

In 2012, the United Kingdom's National Institute for Health Research invited researchers to design a "multicomponent primary care package" for parents of young infants. One aspect of the project was to determine if behavioral interventions promoting consolidated sleep for infants six months or younger improved maternal and infant health. This led to a major systematic review of clinical trials, analyses, and studies on intervention strategies like controlled crying. The research concluded that "these strategies have not been shown to decrease infant crying, prevent sleep and behavioral problems in later childhood, or protect against postnatal depression." It went on to say that intervention strategies applied before six months of age "risk unintended outcomes, including increased amounts of problem crying, premature cessation of breastfeeding, worsened maternal anxiety, and, if the infant is required to sleep either day or night in a room separate from the caregiver, an increased risk of Sudden Infant Death Syndrome."[166]

Ultimately, according to the study, the belief that behavioral interventions in the first few months provide any positive outcome "is historically constructed, overlooks feeding problems, and biases interpretation of data."

Judging by their behavior, infants and children are more content sleeping and waking on their own time and in the company of others, which enhances their feelings of safety, security, and being protected.

Obviously, if an infant's sleep personality naturally lends itself to consolidated sleep at an earlier age, then parents may benefit by it and possibly get more sleep. However, forcing an infant to consolidate sleep does not provide an advantage to the infant. I recognize that parents have every right to make up their own minds as to what they need or want, but we should be clear about whose interest is being served when choosing to sleep train.

---------------- ☽ ----------------

## So-Called "Sleep Problems"

It is hard to ascertain exactly how many infants have what is considered a "sleep problem" in Western society, as it depends on how one defines a "sleep problem," and who is doing the defining. Roughly speaking, somewhere between 40–60% of Western babies are said to have sleep problems in need of solving. My contention is that there is actually nothing wrong with most babies, but, rather, something wrong with the sleep model that is being culturally imposed on them, and the set of expectations it produces.

While most babies do not have sleep problems to solve, their parents do. Parents have the problem of thinking something must be wrong if their baby won't sleep alone or until the morning. They try to impose a model of sleep for which infants are not designed, especially the breastfeeding infant. Western cultures in particular have all but pathologized the natural sleep patterns of breastfeeding infants. An infant's most important job in the first year of life is to wake up all night to breastfeed. It is sad that babies are essentially being victimized simply for being babies and crying when nobody is there to nurture or feed them, a behavior that evolved specifically to retrieve the caregiver on whose body the infant depends for survival.

And do remember this: infants do NOT develop mature sleep in anything resembling a linear fashion. How any individual infant or child develops their sleeping pattern has no template. Infants are all different. But you will save yourself a great deal of disappointment if you avoid getting lulled into thinking that your infant or toddler is finally sleeping through the night. With the way things most often go, he or she will suddenly not be sleeping through the night anymore.

Here's why. As babies mature, their cognitive abilities and executive functioning begins to permit them to make connections between cause and effect, or to imagine the possible negative or scary consequences of things they see during the day, in books you read to them, or on the television. They come to see the possibility that something or somebody could hurt them, or some big sharp-toothed animal or cartoon character might "eat them." They become shy and not so willing to let themselves be handled by strangers, which is good, or may suddenly not be as gregarious in the presence of other people. They may even get a bit more clingy than they were before. After all, as my good friend Dr. Melvin Konner's book *The Evolution of Childhood* reminds us, it's dangerous to be an infant.[167]

The fact that they can be more fearful is generally in their best interest. This is evidence that their brain is becoming more imaginative, flexible, complex, intellectual, and integrated, and they are coming to understand that the world contains dangers that must be avoided.

That babies may go back and forth in their willingness to sleep through the night is a natural and appropriate process of physical, psychological, and cognitive systems developing not necessarily at the same rate or degrees of maturity. It is a reflection of the infants having more complex thoughts and learning to evaluate, make decisions, and think about what could happen, thus making skills and self-regulation seemingly vary from week to week or sometimes from day to day. That is why, as infants get beyond the first year, you may find the child needs to be even closer to you than when they were younger.

Keep in mind that all human beings have their own unique sleep personalities, too, and no two humans (adult or infant) are the same. Most often, infants wake up because it is in their best interest to do so, as their neurobiology is not designed for sustained, deeper sleep before at least six months of age. They

# Is Swaddling a Safe Way to Help Babies Sleep?

The purpose of swaddling a baby is to reduce the frequency of nighttime arousals, which, as I hope you have learned by now, is not actually a safe goal for your infant, at least in the first six months of life. Swaddling simply pushes the notion that we want babies to sleep through the night before they are ready, which cuts down on breastfeeding and, according to at least one study, increases overall risk of SIDS.[168]

Swaddling also stops infants from using their arms, which can be dangerous in the event that something falls onto or in front of their face. Leaving them unswaddled allows them to swat at obstructive items, or to simply have their arms free to protect themselves. Swaddling is particularly dangerous if infants are positioned either on their stomach or side (although an infant should always be placed his or her back to sleep). Based on four studies, it appears that consideration should also be given to the infant's age. The limited evidence we have suggests that swaddling risk increases with age and is associated with a twofold risk of SIDS for infants aged greater than six months.

may appear not to wake up as often when next to their mothers, but in actuality, they wake up more. In these instances, however, they do not necessarily alert the mother, as they are soothed by the simple exchange of sensory information—smelling her milk, hearing her breath, and feeling her body movements and rhythms.

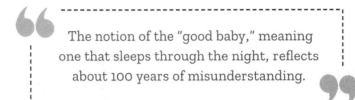

> The notion of the "good baby," meaning one that sleeps through the night, reflects about 100 years of misunderstanding.

The notion of the "good baby," meaning one that sleeps through the night, reflects about 100 years of misunderstanding regarding how our babies should and actually do sleep. The circumstances in which humans evolved favored babies that wake during the night. In the past, nighttime separation from the mother would lead to almost certain death by predators, so babies who cried and successfully retrieved their missing caregivers would, naturally, survive. Personally, if we needed to worry about what any particular baby does, I would worry about the babies who passively accept sleeping alone since it is in their best interest to protest such an arrangement. I might also be concerned about the baby not waking throughout the night to breastfeed, as they could potentially be in danger and fail to realize it or raise the alarm.

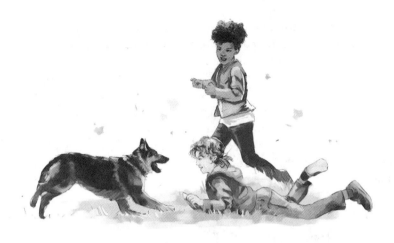

## CHAPTER 11

# Cosleeping in the Long Term

### Lasting Effects on Your Baby

It has never been proven, nor is it even probable, that sleeping in the same room or bed with your baby has any kind of negative long-term effects, provided that the relationships between those involved are healthy and all bedsharing is being done safely. Rather, throughout the years, researchers have found that cosleeping can help a child develop positive qualities, such as more confidence in one's own sexual and gender identities, more comfort with physical affection, a more positive and optimistic attitude about life, more innovativeness, and a comfort with being alone as a toddler.[169]

One major epidemiological study of families living on a military base, wherein one of the married partners is called off for service, showed that it is typical for children to begin to sleep with the remaining parent. Contrary to what the investigators thought they would find, in the sense of psychiatric pathology among the cosleeping children, these children actually required less psychiatric counseling by significant margins compared to children who continued to sleep alone after one of the parents left. The cosleeping children also received higher positive evaluations of their daily behavior from their teachers.[170]

A survey of college-age subjects found that males who coslept with their parents between birth and five years of age had significantly higher self-esteem and experienced less guilt and anxiety. Cosleeping is an important part of the loving, supportive environment that parents create for their children, and will, in turn, give them the confidence they need to grow into social, happy, loving adults.[35, 170, 171, 172, 173, 174, 175]

## The Short- and Long-Term Effects of Childhood Cosleeping

| Study | Ages | Characteristics |
|---|---|---|
| Heron (1994) | 18 months–2 years | Fewer tantrums, more in control of emotions, less fearful, happier |
| Goldberg & Keller (2007) | 2 years | More secure being left alone, able to initiate problem solving in the absence of an adult |
| Okami, Wesiner, & Olmstead (2004) | 6 years | Increased cognitive capacity (for bedsharing children specifically) |
| Forbes & Weiss et al (1992) | 2–13 years | Fewer emotional problems, less often enrolled in psychiatric care, higher rankings on behavior by teachers |
| Lewis and Janda (1988) | 18–23 years | Men have higher self esteem, less anxiety and fear; women have higher self esteem and are more comfortable with intimacy |
| Crawford (1994) | 19–23 years | Women have higher self esteem, confidence, and comfort with intimacy |
| Mosenkis (1997) | 19–26 years | Increased optimism about life and position in life, enhanced satisfaction with occupation, closer family proximity and relationships, rate themselves overall happier |

Fig. 5.2 Many scientific studies have proven that cosleeping infants or children reap behavioral, emotional, and intellectual benefits throughout their lives.

While it's nice to be able to cite many research papers that show long-term psychological benefits associated with bedsharing among children and young adults, something is still being missed. Here it is important to remember the main determinant of short-term and long-term bedsharing outcomes, which is the nature of the relationship being brought to the shared sleep space. In other words, obviously children share a certain type of relationship on a 24/7 basis with their parents, and not just at night. If this relationship is loving and caring and respectful during the day (i.e., healthy), then bedsharing children simply get more of what is already good; if the relationship is not so healthy, then obviously at night the children would be getting more of what is already bad for them during the day. It is the nature of this relationship that matters, not just where it plays out.

——————— ❭ ———————

## Naptime Strategies

Most babies don't mind sleeping alone for naps during the day—it's the darkness of nighttime that is intimidating. But it is ideal to avoid isolating babies at any time, even for naps. Putting babies down for a nap has become a unique Western custom, especially the thinking that goes along with it. In reality, letting an infant fall asleep when and where his or her body wants to is a much smarter strategy. The sensory stimulation from the sounds of other people talking, laughing, and moving are actually protective against SIDS, along with the parental vigilance that accompanies it. In accordance with the main theme of this book, even for naps, infants should never sleep outside the supervision of a committed adult.

Try to let your baby nap in a bassinet or crib wherever there are people around, if this is possible. Don't worry about your baby not being able to fall asleep, because most babies can sleep anywhere if they are tired. The old maxim of *Shhhh! The baby is sleeping,* only conditions a baby to sleep lightly and to stir at each extraneous noise. Babies likely feel secure hearing the voices of their siblings and parents while sleeping. The level of normal

# What Other Practices Contribute to an Infant's Health and Safety?

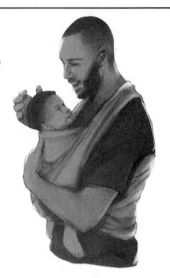

The more you hold, carry, and interact with your baby, the better. Carrying babies in contact with your body contributes greatly to their healthy development. This is especially true when considering the development of your baby's neck muscles, which can be crucial if a baby needs to move his or her head away from something obstructing oxygen flow. Carrying your baby on your hip is a universal carrying pattern that gives your baby a front row seat to all that is going on. Baby-wearing wraps or snuggles made out of cloth are also great. These permit maximum exposure of the baby's face and allow the baby to swivel his or her head and engage with the environment. Baby-wearing promotes incredibly important intellectual and social benefits for infants. Your infant engaging with your friends, family, and relatives, and observing where he or she is and what is happening in the environment around them, is almost like the infant attending school.

If possible, try to cut down on keeping babies in plastic holding or carrying containers, as they have contributed to some infants developing flat heads. Platycephally (flattening) of the head is not necessarily caused by infants sleeping on their backs, but rather by how long they lean their heads against hard objects. This is especially a concern with what I call "transformer baby furniture," or furniture that can change into many different pieces, keeping the baby's head against a hard surface for hours.

Parents should also make taking care of themselves a priority, so they are ready to respond to their baby's needs. Good sleep habits—avoiding caffeine, not using electronics before bed, and, as difficult as it sounds as a new parent, trying to turn in and wake up at the same time every day—can all help you get more rest. Try sleeping while the baby sleeps, skipping household chores, sharing nighttime baby duties, asking friends and family for help, and taking advantage of parental leave from work.

noises in a household assures a level of arousal in your baby that is probably just about right for the safest possible sleep.

When out of the house visiting friends and family, I hear that parents often put their baby down for a nap on top of an adult bed. Sometimes they will place pillows on either side of the baby to keep the infant from rolling off the bed. However, we have learned that pillows pose a suffocation risk. So, what do you do in this situation?

First of all, I still would not recommend putting a baby "down for a nap" in a separate room, but instead let the baby sleep in the context of the people and activities in his or her environment. That being said, if you absolutely must have your baby nap somewhere less disruptive, there are still relatively safe options.

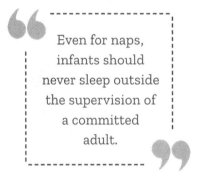

Even for naps, infants should never sleep outside the supervision of a committed adult.

A newborn, if placed in the middle of a firm adult bed, will not move around very much. I don't like the idea of newborns being alone in an adult bed, but as long as there are no extra pillows or blankets near the baby, and the duvet is not too fluffy, that should work just fine without the need for pillows to keep the baby in place.

A four- or five-month-old baby is much more mobile, which can pose a serious falling or wedging risk if a parent or responsible adult is not there, depending on the bed and the furniture around the bed. In this case, you can place the infant on the floor on a sheet or a clean towel, on his or her back, in a wide, clear space. The infant must be on a firm surface, without any pillows or extra objects around. I am personally a fan of the HALO SleepSack®, (basically a wearable blanket) to make a cozy, convenient sleep space without loose blankets.

If your baby is too mobile and you're worried about him or her roaming about the room, it might be useful to invest in a portable play pen or baby gates (without bars where a baby could get stuck).

One more note: if the infant absolutely must nap in another room, use a spare baby monitor in the opposite way you would normally use it. Turn the speakers around and broadcast the sounds and noises made in the active portion of the house into the room where your baby is sleeping. This will provide background noise to help your baby enjoy healthy arousals, and otherwise sleep in a way that is the most natural for his or her body. Remember, at least 100 years of developmental science tells us that babies have a healthier reaction to sound than to silence. Piping in human voices is especially reassuring for infants, like a "life force" inviting a physiological response. Feeding these sounds into the baby's room is actually more proactive and protective than using a monitor to hear the baby, because it can provide, to a lesser degree, many of the same biological and developmental benefits as the act of cosleeping.

)

## Cosleeping While Traveling

During the first few years of life, you will find your infant or child will feel especially reassured sleeping in your company when away from home. Many parents who do not ordinarily practice cosleeping permit it while traveling.

The problem is, however, that this change in routine seems to constitute a higher risk of SIDS. That is, babies between two and four months of age who sleep alone while traveling, when they ordinarily do not sleep alone, have a slight increased risk of dying from SIDS, and vice versa. A baby who does not ordinarily breastsleep, but does so while sleeping away from home, is at an increased risk of SIDS, because he or she is in a new sleep environment. The bottom line: perhaps it is best while traveling to mimic as closely as possible what you ordinarily do at home. If you breastsleep, breastsleep; if you sleep apart, sleep apart.

Keep in mind that if you are breastsleeping while traveling, you need to ensure that the breastsleeping setup is safe for your baby (see Part 4: How to Cosleep). When you are traveling or on vacation, risk factors that can endanger your baby are still present. These risks may even be increased, so it pays to be extra careful regarding where and how your baby sleeps while traveling.

# Weaning in a Breastsleeping Situation

It is a process to wean a baby who has slept next to you and breastfed on demand from birth. Like all infant caregiving practices, choosing when and how to wean your baby while breastsleeping is a decision only you (and your partner) can make.

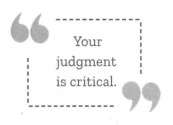

Your judgment is critical.

Some babies may have difficulty adjusting to less breastfeeding. One potential strategy to reduce night breastfeeding is to breastfeed your baby more during the day. While bedsharing, placing a solid, non-cloth barrier (especially not a pillow) between your breast and the baby can sometimes reduce the infant's detection of milk nearby and eliminate some feedings, as can simply placing the baby in a crib in your room, or next to you in a bassinet. These options can work for some babies, but certainly not all.

If your baby is crying to be fed, your partner can walk with the baby to help them learn a new association. Your partner's role in weaning a baby from night feedings can be very rewarding, and can help to strengthen your partner's attachment relationship with the baby. I used to dance with my son when he was fussy, because the swaying and rhythms would put him to sleep, and for me it was fun and good exercise!

Trusting and using your own judgment and experience with your baby is always important, since you know more than anyone about your baby's history, preferences, personality, temperament, and idiosyncrasies. Everyone has an opinion on what you should do with your baby, and they are not afraid to tell you about it, but your judgment is critical. The reality is that every baby will give you different insights as to what works best for them, and only them, and it won't always be the same from baby to baby, as many parents quickly discover. As with the decision to cosleep or breastsleep, the decision to wean has to be made by you, with careful, thorough consideration of your own—and your entire family's—particular needs.

## Deciding How Long to Cosleep

Keep in mind that it is entirely up to you to determine the best time for your family to stop bedsharing or roomsharing, assuming that the relationship you share is healthy. This decision is similar to, say, what age you feel comfortable with your teenager starting to date or getting their driver's license. There is really no hard and fast cut-off, just as long as everyone is happy with the arrangements.

In most cultures around the world, people sleep in the same room with their different family members in one form or another throughout their lives. The idea that there are cut-offs is another Western cultural meme, and it varies based on who is making the decision and how any given parental behavior or caregiving activity resonates with all the relationships and unique psychological states involved. The idea that there are specific cut-off times for sleeping arrangements is certainly not mandated by any scientific finding. Again, this is about your relationship with your infant or child, and with your partner, and what they might be feeling too. Someone else's preference or answer has nothing to do with what your own decision will be as to how long to bedshare, and as I will keep repeating, these are all relational issues. Just as we should not judge what others do, we should also not be judged for what we decide in the context of these experiences.

It is important to remember that there is absolutely nothing wrong with deciding that you are ready to have your child sleep in his or her own room; the key is to trust your knowledge of yourself and your child in deciding how best to do it. You know both yourself and your baby better than anyone, so I have no doubt that it is you and not any external professional that will know how best to do this.

# How Do I Get My Baby out of My Bed?

Ahh, a common question I am asked to respond to. I have spent most of my life providing parents with good scientific reasons to take their babies to bed with them, should they feel comfortable doing so. I am less concerned about finding ways to separate families at night because, as I have said before, you are the most familiar with your baby, and hence should be in the best position to figure this one out yourself. But I will try to give you some general ideas.

For example, some parents try making bedtime full of stories and rituals unique to your child, or offer a doll or favorite object as a sleeping companion. Easing the child from the bed by having them sleep on the floor or a mat next to the parent's bed, or on a separate cot or bed within the same room, can help them feel more comfortable moving to their own sleeping space.

Merely stressing the excitement of a new room or having special privileges as an older child may be enough. For some toddlers or children, a fancy-dancy toy-like bed, or some sort of themed bed could work. Or, putting your toddler in a room with a sibling can help to make the transition easier. Changing routines is a necessary part of growing up, and the transition away from cosleeping can still be a positive experience for your child.

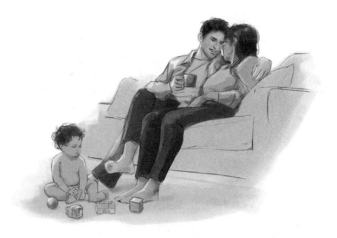

CHAPTER 12

# Dispelling Myths

## "Cosleeping Will Change Your Relationship With Your Child"

I often hear concerns that the relationship a parent has with their child is somehow going to change if they begin cosleeping. This is simply not true. Sleeping arrangements do not alter a relationship, but they reflect the nature of it. Don't forget that the child-parent relationship is already being shared before going to bed. In other words, sleeping arrangements generally reflect and sometimes strengthen, contribute to, or exaggerate the nature of the relationship that already exists, whether good or less optimal.

If the nature of a relationship is very good during the day, cosleeping simply makes whatever is already good just as good, or even better, at night. I spoke more about this in the previous chapter.

In contrast, if a parent is depressed or is resentful of the infant during the day, these same dynamics will impact the child negatively during the night; if these negatively inclined parents choose to cosleep, it could lead to more neglectful cosleeping practices.

Parents should keep in mind that if they are struggling mentally or emotionally, it is sometimes best for their own health to allow a little space from the infant, especially at night when it is time to rest and recharge. Ultimately, taking care of your own mental health will positively affect your ability to care for and develop a relationship with your infant. But, that said, cosleeping can be a wonderful way for content and affectionate parents to continue to deepen the bond with their child during the night.

———————— ❯ ————————

## "Cosleeping Will Get in the Way of Your Child's Independence"

Ultimately, this is false, but cosleeping will likely delay your baby's willingness to be alone when they sleep, and their willingness to self-soothe. Sometimes parents are under the mistaken impression that if they don't train their babies to sleep by themselves, somehow some developmental or social skill will be kept from them later in life. This is not true, as we explored in Chapter 11. They also worry that their babies won't exhibit good sleep patterns as adults. This is not true, either. In reality, there aren't any scientific studies that have shown any benefit whatsoever to sleeping through the night at infantile ages, or to sleeping through the night uninterrupted even as an adult. And, as mentioned previously, early consolidation of infant sleep will conflict with or make less likely more optimal breastfeeding.

Some people confuse an infant's willingness to soothe him- or herself back to sleep as a sign of independence, autonomy, or confidence. In reality, life-long self-sufficiency has absolutely nothing to do with the age at which infants put themselves back to sleep without a parent or loved one, i.e., "self soothe." Studies by psychologists Meret Keller and Wendy Goldberg have shown that children who routinely sleep with their parents actually become more independent socially and psychologically. Contrary to the popular belief that solitary sleep produces confident and secure children, while cosleeping infants will grow to be clingy and overly dependent, cosleeping toddlers are actually able to be alone and solve problems on their own better than solitary sleepers.[176] These were the first actual studies addressing this popular misconception.

In this research, Keller and Goldberg carefully defined what they mean by "independence" and, with this definition, they provide us with a solid starting point for further examination. When compared to solitary-sleeping children, the cosleeping children in their sample tended to make friends more easily, could initiate problem solving more independently, and could be by themselves with less stress. Other studies have shown that cosleeping children are significantly less likely to throw temper tantrums.[170, 171, 177, 178] A cross-cultural comparison of Norwegian children and Sámi children, indigenous to Norway and Sweden, challenges the belief that solitary sleep is positively correlated with independence. More Sámi children slept with their parents than Norwegian children, yet Sámi children were observed to be significantly less demanding of their parents' attention during play than their Norwegian counterparts.[179]

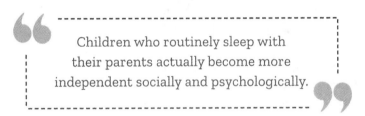

Children who routinely sleep with their parents actually become more independent socially and psychologically.

Another way to consider the question of independence is to ask whether we really want our children to be independent from us, and, if so, what exactly do we mean? When a father worries that his four-month-old infant son is too "soft" and "dependent," as one father said to me, does that mean he will feel happy if he sees his 14-year-old son seeking advice from young male peers rather than from him? I doubt it.

British psychiatrist Dr. Jeremy Holmes points out that "Autonomy in the context of psychotherapy implies taking control of one's own life…[but] emotional autonomy does not mean isolation or avoidance of dependency. On the contrary, the lonely schizoid individual who preserves his 'independence' at all costs may well be in a state of emotional heteronomy unable to bear closeness with another person because of inner dread and confusion. The emotionally autonomous individual does not suppress her feelings, including her need for dependence, but takes cognizance of them, ruling rather than being ruled by them."[180]

The idea that you should leave your baby alone during the night, an idea believed by many, is completely antithetical to 100 years of information on what is involved in facilitating the development of empathy and autonomy, as well as the ability to be alone when one needs to be and the ability to interrelate and to become interdependent with others. As you begin to know your child better and identify your priorities as a parent, most of you will want to guide your children toward these goals. One way we can help our children achieve these goals is to maximize the attention and protection we offer them at night by sleeping close to them.

---

## "Cosleeping Will Negatively Affect Your Relationship With Your Partner"

Because your family is unique, it is impossible to say with certainty how cosleeping will affect your relationship with your partner, but I can say the following: New parents are faced with numerous challenges and rewards as they adjust to their roles as mothers and fathers, and developing a sleeping pattern that works for your family is just one challenge among many.

There are several things to keep in mind as you develop your cosleeping patterns, but cosleeping doesn't have to affect tenderness and closeness between spouses.

With the baby in the bed, you can still talk, touch, laugh, massage, and otherwise enjoy the connection with your partner. As far as intercourse goes, as long as the infant is in a safe place near your bed, I don't believe any infant or child has been psychologically damaged by hearing the love-making of their parents, although it might be advised not to vocalize too enthusiastically for fear of frightening your child. I would suggest not to have sex when your baby is in bed with you, but that precaution is fairly intuitive. Beyond that, it is really up to you to decide what you are comfortable doing while the baby is in the room.

Intimacy may have to be less spontaneous—for instance, you may need to start scheduling time together when someone else can tend to the baby, or move the baby into a crib or bassinet for a few hours after they fall asleep, with some form of baby monitor on hand—but intimacy does not, by any means, have to be eliminated, and can strengthen your bond as co-parents.

Ultimately, every couple is different and the way each family works is different, but parenting is best done as a team—with both individuals fully committed to raising children in the same way. Like most other domains of married or partnered life, agreements and compromises are very important. Hence, it is always best for parents or partners to discuss their goals, concerns, and philosophies, and to strive toward a consensus on raising their child. Whatever the challenges might be, they are easier solved if both partners agree on what experiences they want to share.

The best research thus far on this complex issue, involving an analysis of the criss-crossing relationships and psychologies unique to each family, does not point to any simple answer for how sleeping arrangements affect marital relationships.[172, 173, 181] If there is any singular perspective offered by these works, it is that there is no blanket statement that may be said about how cosleeping will affect your relationship.

───────── ❱ ─────────

## "Cosleeping Creates a Bad Habit"

This ubiquitous warning is based on subjective and perceived values; it is a personal judgment by someone who evaluates cosleeping very differently than you might. One parent's "bad habit" is another parent's greatest joy—the privilege of being close to their beloved infant. As a father of a cosleeping infant and toddler, I enjoyed every minute I was able to be close to my son in bed. Time spent cosleeping may be a family's most treasured time together, and for most parents and babies (though maybe not all), breastsleeping and bedsharing is natural and enjoyable.

Like adults, infants and children will be reluctant to give up something that feels right to them. That said, any human habit can be broken, and the way new sleeping arrangements are introduced depends on the personalities of the parents and children involved and the special characteristics of the family.

You will find that, like all matters that are relational, the relationship you develop with your own child requires trade-offs. For example, if you choose to routinely cosleep all night every night with your child, you will derive great feelings and memories from the experience. Along with that, your child may develop a more permanent capacity for self-sufficiency, resilience, comfort with affection, and the ability to be alone when necessary.

The trade-off is that you and your child may have less consolidated sleep. You should also be prepared for the possibility that, when you are ready to "wean" your child from your room or bed, they may not be on the same timetable as you. One study found that, compared with solitary sleepers from birth, infants who cosleep from birth either learn or accept sleeping alone about a year later than infants who have no choice but to sleep alone. Even so, eventually separate sleep will not be a problem for your child, just as with children who sleep alone from an early age.[176]

In every relationship we gain and give up things, and often make compromises. In the end, only the cosleeping participants can know if the trade-off balance translates to a bad habit, but, for many families, the benefits far outweigh the costs.

## "Babies Need Silence to Fall Asleep"

Most people have experienced someone saying "Shush! I just put the baby down for a nap," but, in actuality, infants can fall asleep in the middle of a rock concert if they need to. Even though it is generally thought that babies need silence to sleep, you might notice that infants sometimes fall asleep quickly in the context of a lot of family noise and excitement. This is a way for infants to regulate feeling over-stimulated—they simply go to sleep.

As I discussed earlier, as long as the stimulation is not too overwhelming, babies typically feel more secure hearing that a caregiver is nearby. At least 50 years of human development research shows that babies respond positively when they "feel" that they are not alone, through physical and psychological sensory signals (voices or other sounds, sights, smells, touches, and movement).

Some parents may choose to put the infant down for a nap in a separate room with the door closed, where sensory access between the baby and the parents (and other family members) is not possible or likely.

Admittedly—and I must laugh at myself for this—before I came to study infant sleep, I would often carefully lie my baby down to sleep in a separate space. I would walk away slowly, step by step, putting my foot down gently and hoping that the floor would not creak. When it did, my son would open his eyes, letting me know to "forget it, you've been caught." And I was!

My recommendation today is never to close the door to a baby's room since babies find sleep when they need it, and they were not designed to sleep in complete social and sensory isolation. A silent environment for the infant does nothing but potentially condition the baby to only be able to fall asleep in silence.

Some parents find it comforting to put some kind of baby monitor in the room. This is fine, but, as I have mentioned before, a more appropriate use would be to turn the amplifiers around to broadcast family voices into the baby's room. If the baby must be in a room by him- or herself, letting the baby hear the chatter of parents and siblings, rather than the other way around, can potentially be protective against SIDS. If using monitors in the usual way (to hear your baby) is very important to you, leaving a radio on near the baby with a mix of talking, music, or other varied sounds may have a similar effect.

Human voices are reassuring to infants, but it is always possible that a loud TV or an active herd of siblings could make it difficult for the baby to sleep if they are not very tired. Ultimately, it's important that noise levels are kept consistent. If your child falls asleep to noise, hearing less noise—or, likewise, a sudden loud noise—might wake them. Either way, it's generally hard to keep a baby awake if he or she is sleepy.

Only you can be the judge of how intrusive the noise level

might be for your baby. When in doubt, just keep in mind that infants can protect themselves from excessive stimulation, but what they cannot protect themselves from is too little stimulation.

——————— ❭ ———————

# "We Won't Get a Good Night's Sleep"

The truthfulness of this statement depends, in part, on exactly how parents define a "good night's sleep," and whether cosleeping or breastsleeping is a choice made by the parents or a situation they feel was imposed on them by their child's inability to sleep alone. This varies for different families. A research paper from years ago argued that there are important differences in parents' evaluations of their cosleeping behavior based on whether or not they are cosleeping in response to ongoing "sleep problems" their children are having, or if they have chosen to cosleep due to their own philosophies or emotional needs.[182] The former type of cosleeping was called by the authors, "reactionary cosleeping," which was evaluated more negatively. Not unexpectedly, intentional cosleeping was evaluated much more positively by the parents.

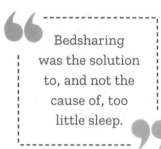

Bedsharing was the solution to, and not the cause of, too little sleep.

Generally, bedsharing mother-infant pairs have many more brief, transient arousals, and the infants tend to breastfeed much more frequently; but the perception by these mothers of their own sleep in these cases can, nonetheless, be very positive. In fact, research has shown that bedsharing was the solution to, and not the cause of, too little sleep.[36, 183]

According to mothers themselves, the choice to breastsleep with infants tends to promote a longer, more restful night's sleep for both babies and parents alike. A baby sleeping in a separate room, in order to elicit a feeding from the mother, needs to cry. This generally makes the baby less calm and more excited, even before breastfeeding begins. Reflecting on their observation that crying is a "late" signal given by a baby in need of a breastfeed, the Breastfeeding Subcommittee of the AAP pointed out that infants show a number of signals—such as sucking, wiggling, placing alternating hands on their mother's chest, and sucking their own fists—which provide ample time for the mother, if already in proximity, to initiate a feed before the infant cries.

We witnessed this frequently in our laboratory studies when separate-sleeping, breastfeeding mothers had a hard time putting their infant back down in a crib in another room. As soon as the infants hit the crib mattress after a feed, they would typically cry. Then up the baby would come for another feeding attempt, only to be placed back in the crib. We were sure from what we repeatedly saw that the babies were not fussing because they needed more milk, but because they needed to be held and to be in contact with their mother.

Compared to breastsleeping mothers, it typically took significantly longer for separate-sleeping, breastfeeding mothers to put their baby down, meaning that Mom had to stay awake longer, too. Even if a bedsharing baby wakes to breastfeed more often than if he or she were in a separate room, Mom doesn't have to get out of bed, doesn't have to disturb her partner, and barely has to wake herself to feed and soothe her infant.

In fact, we quantified this observation in our laboratory study of bedsharing and solitary-sleeping mother-infant dyads. Bedsharing mothers received more sleep, in minutes, than did solitary-sleeping mothers.[33] Also, interestingly, mothers underestimated how many times they woke to breastfeed by as much as 50%, and 84% of bedsharing mothers said that they had "good" or "enough" sleep, while only 64% of the solitary-sleeping moms said that they had "good" or "enough" sleep. Some mothers choose to breastsleep because that is the only way they can get enough sleep.

# Part 6

## Final Thoughts

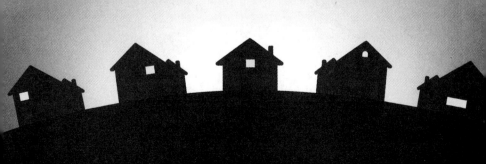

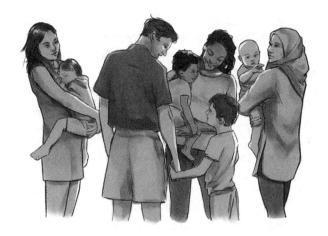

CHAPTER 13

# Is the Tide Turning?

I think it's quite possible for the United States and other countries with similar sleep safety guidelines to remove the stigma surrounding all forms of cosleeping, including breastsleeping. Indeed, we have already made a surprising amount of progress starting from the very beginning of pediatric sleep studies, hardly more than 40 years ago.

Back then, it was simply assumed that we in Western industrialized societies were the only humans on the planet who knew best what babies need at night and how to care for them. We never thought to use an anthropological lens to look worldwide at how most human infants sleep. Had we looked, we would have found that infants universally sleep next to at least one caregiver—usually the breastfeeding mother.

Early Western pediatric sleep scientists also assumed that infant formula was the best and most convenient way to feed a baby. Formula (and cow's milk) contains more calories than human milk and is not easily digested. For this reason, formula-fed babies do not need to be fed as often as breastfed babies, promoting consolidated, uninterrupted sleep.

This uninterrupted sleep is what early pediatric sleep scientists chose to strive for. Their guidelines were unfortunately based not on infant needs, but on the cultural ideal of the "good baby" who bottle-feeds and sleeps through the night without crying. Mainly, babies were supposed to be placed alone in a crib in a separate room and taught to self-soothe. Of course, now we know how wrong that ideal is. This is where I see the most progress in today's safe sleep recommendations.

Formula-feeding and deep, uninterrupted sleep have been proven to make it easier for babies to die from SIDS. Current infant sleep guidelines have finally admitted that breastfeeding throughout the first year of life can protect against SIDS and provide many other exceptional benefits. Amazingly, the American Academy of Pediatrics also acknowledges that, when parents fall asleep while feeding their babies, it is "less hazardous to fall asleep with the infant in the adult bed than on a sofa or armchair...."[184]

Perhaps due to these slow policy changes, combined with modern research showing the protective benefits of breastsleeping, many countries have seen an increase in bedsharing rates. Even back in 2008, Dr. Peter Blair noted a significant increase in the popularity of cosleeping around the world:

"In England, almost half of all neonates [infants less than four weeks old] bedshare at some time with their parent; 1/5 of infants are brought into the parental bed on a regular basis over the first year of life. Similar or higher rates of bedsharing at three months of age have recently been reported in other European countries; Ireland (21%), Germany (23%), Italy (24%), Scotland (25%), Austria (30%), Denmark (39%), Sweden (65%). Even in countries where bedsharing is uncommon, such as [the Netherlands], Norway, and the U.S., all have reported an increase in the prevalence of bedsharing in the last decade."[185]

Even better, research from many fields is currently coalescing to make powerful arguments against an over-simplified, uniform approach to sleep safety recommendations. As of 2019, two important papers[1, 186] are helping turn the tide by arguing that bedsharing does not cause SIDS. They implore medical authorities, including the AAP, to change their negative rhetoric against all bedsharing, acknowledge the diversity of bedsharing, and recognize the crucial importance of respecting and valuing a family's choice to sleep alongside their infant in bed.

That being said, there is still plenty of progress that needs to be made. If we really want to reduce sleep-related infant deaths, we need to be placing a much greater emphasis on a few main points that are currently buried in pediatric recommendations: the reduction of formula-feeding, the reduction of smoking in the home, education on the dangers of sofas or recliners for sleep, and, of course, safe bedsharing practices.

Any responsible public health official should be teaching parents how to safely bedshare. Their goal should not be disseminating doctrine or telling you how you should raise your children, but rather coaching families based on their individual circumstances and goals. If parents are going to bedshare regardless of what they are told (which they are), then it is the health expert's responsibility to help them do it safely.

---

*"What is clear is that the negative rhetoric that eliminates any hope of honest, bi-directional conversations between bedsharing parents and their health providers must cease and be replaced by an emphasis on the magnitude of risk surrounding unsafe sleeping practices involving alcohol, drugs, and sofas or chairs, establishing a more coordinated approach with other public health strategists on how best to care for the infants as well as to keep them safe."*

—DR. KATHLEEN A. MARINELLI, ET AL.[1]

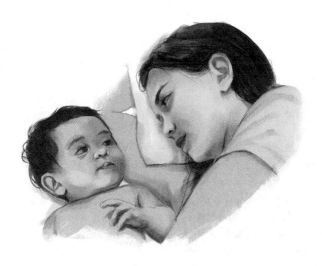

CHAPTER 14

# The State of Our Parenting

## Where We Stand and Where Our Babies Sleep

*"The great enemy of truth is very often not the lie—deliberate, contrived, and dishonest—but the myth—persistent, persuasive, and unrealistic. Too often we hold fast to the clichés of our forebears. We subject all facts to a prefabricated set of interpretations. We enjoy the comfort of opinion without the discomfort of thought."*

—PRESIDENT JOHN F. KENNEDY[187]

I never could have imagined that any U.S. government institution or insular medical group in modern society would want to eradicate the occurrence of mothers sleeping with their infants.

Eliminating bedsharing will fail, of course, as it already has. It is an attempt to override appropriate human behavior and biology. The fact is that a mother sleeping with her baby is an inherent human right, not an unhealthy condition or something mothers do to be cool.

Mother-infant cosleeping, in all its diverse forms, is a universal human experience and a biological necessity. It will not be suppressed by cultural messages. No group, especially one funded by the public, has the right to tell parents not to cosleep, except when it is being done unsafely.

Unfortunately, one fact remains. As previously argued,[2, 8, 116, 137] there are not many places where the social values, expectations, and preferences of the Western industrial world are more strongly reflected than in the clinical models of what "normal, healthy" sleep and "normal, healthy" sleeping arrangements should look like in the first year of an infant's life.[98, 188]

Considering how the misguided sleep safety campaigns, however well-intentioned, are spreading from the U.S. to many other cultures, it is evident that a more inclusive science and more effective safety strategy are being held hostage by the views and opinions of a small group of people and their personal ideologies. Most research papers are only interested in proving and confirming what this small group believes to be true, while discarding any possibility of studying what makes breastsleeping safe and why the overwhelming number of breastsleeping babies not only live, but flourish.

The tactics being used by the U.S. government and hospitals around the country are shamefully one-sided, with parents being shown videos of the publicly approved version of "safe infant sleep." In some cases, they are expected to sign statements implying that they may be subject to prosecution if anything happens to their infant in a bedsharing environment. It is important to determine ahead of time if the hospital you have in mind has such policies and whether you can accept being treated this way.

Some U.S. hospitals no longer permit an infant to be in bed with the mother at all, even when the mother is awake. Fewer hospitals seem comfortable encouraging any kind of sustained contact between a mother and her infant, despite strong evidence that it may enhance successful breastfeeding and augment the number of months that mothers breastfeed their infants. The heavy emphasis on denying spontaneous contact between mother and infant leads me to believe that if these guidelines, along with recommendations against breastsleeping, are widely adopted, there will be a widespread negative impact on breastfeeding rates and on the natural joy that mothers and fathers experience when in contact with their baby.

The lack of regard for parents and for legitimate scientists demonstrates just how problematic public health approaches and policies can be when exclusively based on political or cultural ideologies. All scientific data and perspectives should be considered, exchanged, integrated, and shared openly with mutual respect.

Going forward, we also need to seriously confront and acknowledge the larger socio-political challenges (hidden as they are) that shape anti-bedsharing recommendations. This part of the conversation involves seeking answers for why the safety of bedsharing, and infant mortality in general, varies so much between and within socioeconomic and racial sub-groups.

Environments of infant sleep matter greatly, but they are part of a larger system of family relationships and communal life. These systems are defined and constrained by access to resources, leading to conditions of chronic stress for minority or marginalized sub-groups, which in turn create inter-generational injuries in the form of excessive infant health problems. Unfortunately, the misleading classification of infant deaths related to these issues allows our society to point to bedsharing as the cause, and to gloss over or dismiss the real, more problematic roots.[2, 189]

Putting the blame for chaotic cosleeping deaths on bedsharing itself, rather than on the conditions and diverse social circumstances that make the practice safe for some subgroups, but not for others, is morally and scientifically wrong. Reducing the broad range of bedsharing behaviors to a simplistic, universally-dangerous act fails to take into account much of what has been learned in the developmental and evolutionary sciences regarding the critical long-term and short-term health effects of cosleeping. This includes increased physical contact that confers potential genetic benefits to infants and their future children—a benefit that had not been identified before this last decade.[5]

Attempts to eradicate bedsharing—calling it inherently unsafe without considering the modifiable factors that can make it so—is a mistake that can easily be corrected by educating those communities whose babies are most at risk.

If breastfeeding promotion activities are directed toward communities where bedsharing deaths are disproportionately high, increased breastfeeding rates will put into place a suite of powerful behavioral and physiological safeguards to protect at-risk infants, reducing sleep-related deaths while improving the health of mothers and infants in general. In order for this to happen, we need public health organizations to shift their efforts and funding toward promoting breastfeeding, and away from anti-bedsharing messages.

Unfortunately, nothing will change if breastsleeping parents remain silent. The more parents that are honest about where their babies actually sleep, the sooner we will get accurate numbers of how many parents do, in fact, bedshare. Dr. Kendall-Tackett's research[37] reveals this startling statistic: 70% of her sample of bedsharing mothers were less likely to tell their health care providers about where their babies end the night than those who roomshare. I think it's time to start sharing the truth.

I would encourage you to be open with your family and friends, and especially your pediatrician. You might handle that conversation by explaining that you are thoroughly informed on the benefits and the risks of all sleeping arrangements, and that you feel secure in your decision about what arrangement is best for you and your family. You can tell them you value their thoughts and are open to discussing your decisions, with the hope that it can be a respectful, two-way conversation. This kind of conversation is what the Academy of Breastfeeding Medicine has officially recommended in their most recent bedsharing protocol.[190] More specific information about this, and recommended approaches to the bedsharing issue, can also be found in a new paper written by five internationally-recognized SIDS, infant sleep, and breastfeeding experts.[1]

I know sharing your viewpoint will not always be easy, since being open carries the risk of lectures and criticism. However, if physicians were to realize how many parents are bedsharing, whether breastsleeping or not, I think they would be more aware of the important and beneficial functions breastsleeping has played throughout our evolution, and might come to understand why the practice cannot and will not be eradicated.

In sum, I wrote this book to assure you that if you are able to arrange a safe bedsharing environment for your infant, following my own, your own, or the safety tips suggested by La Leche League International in their book *Sweet Sleep*, bedsharing can be a positive, safe, and affirming experience for breastfeeding mothers and infants alike. There is no doubt that we are in a time of transition and that challenges lie ahead, but one thing is for sure. Present recommendations regarding infant sleeping arrangements not only place infants and mothers at odds with their own emotions, but also with their own societies within which emotional behaviors like breastsleeping find expression.

Standing firm as to your right to choose for yourself where your baby sleeps may be challenging, but it is imperative. Speak out and share your views. Physicians, especially, must know how strongly you feel and how common breastsleeping really is. It is no longer acceptable to remain silent while individuals who know nothing about your family continue to endorse a singular, negative, "authoritative" view that dismisses the insights and confidence of other researchers, as well as parents who acquire invaluable knowledge about the unique needs of their own infants and how best to respond to them. Enjoy your baby, celebrate the love you and your family are privileged to enjoy and, by all means, feel comfortable knowing that you will always remain the best judge of what is and is not good for all of you.

# Appendices

# APPENDIX I
# Glossary of Terms

*When it comes to infant sleep arrangements, parents and professionals alike use different phrases interchangeably and confuse related terminology. Here is a glossary of the most common terms so everyone can begin to have conversations using the same language.*

*Note: Because these terms are inter-related, these definitions build upon one another. For this reason, this glossary is not ordered alphabetically.*

<u>Cosleeping:</u> The general term for sleeping within range of detecting the signals from another person, regardless of age. Encompasses roomsharing, separate-surface cosleeping, use of a cosleeping device, same-surface cosleeping, bedsharing, cobedding, and breastsleeping.

<u>Roomsharing:</u> Sleeping in the same room as another person, regardless of age, but on a separate surface. Includes a baby sleeping in a crib or bassinet next to the parent's bed, or in a cosleeping device. Also known as separate-surface cosleeping.

<u>Separate-Surface Cosleeping:</u> Sleeping in the same room as another person, regardless of age, within sensory range of each other, but on a separate surface. Includes a baby sleeping in a crib or bassinet next to the parent's bed or in a cosleeping device. Also known as roomsharing.

<u>Cosleeping Device:</u> A product that allows a baby to sleep in close proximity to his or her parents without being on the same surface. It may attach to or rest beside the bed, or sit on top of the bed. Use of a cosleeping device can be considered roomsharing or separate-surface cosleeping.

<u>Same-Surface Cosleeping:</u> Sleeping on the same surface as another person, regardless of age. Includes sleeping on a bed, on a couch (which is dangerous), or on any other surface. Encompasses cobedding, bedsharing, and breastsleeping.

**Cobedding:** Two bodies of the same size sleeping on the same surface, such as twins sharing a single crib.

**Bedsharing:** Sleeping in the same bed as another person, regardless of age. Includes breastsleeping.

**Breastsleeping:** A primarily breastfed baby sleeping in the same bed as his or her mother in order to facilitate breastfeeding, with the infant lying face-up, in an environment free from all hazardous risk factors.

**Hazardous Risk Factors:** Circumstances that increase the risk of SUID when combined with bedsharing or by themselves—these include sleeping next to an adult who is impaired by alcohol or drugs, smoke exposure, sleeping face-down, sleeping on a sofa with an adult, preterm birth, formula-feeding, and soft bedding (definition from Peter S. Blair, et al., in press[190]).

**Epidemiology:** The study of the distribution, causes, and risk factors of diseases or other health and safety issues within a specified population (definition adapted from *Principles of Epidemiology in Public Health Practice, 3rd Edition*).

**Sudden Unexpected Infant Death (SUID) or
Sudden Unexpected Death in Infancy (SUDI):** The sudden and unexpected death of a baby less than one year old in which the cause was not obvious before investigation. Encompasses both SIDS and SASS.

SUID/SUDI are also broadly defined in the International Classification of Diseases, 10th Revision (ICD-10), as a compilation of classifications that include SIDS, ASSB, and unspecified deaths lacking evidence to be called SIDS.

**Sudden Infant Death Syndrome (SIDS):** The sudden and unexplained death of a baby younger than one year of age, without a known cause even after a complete investigation (definition from the National Institute of Child Health and Human Development). See page 67 to explore the difference between SIDS and SASS in the context of bedsharing.

**Sleep Associated Suffocation and Strangulation (SASS) or Accidental Suffocation or Strangulation in Bed (ASSB):** The accidental sleep-related death of a baby by suffocation or strangulation, often due to unsafe cosleeping environments.

SASS (term proposed by Melissa Bartick and Linda J. Smith[191]) is more commonly referred to as ASSB, which is how it appears in the International Classification of Diseases, 10th Revision (ICD-10). Confusingly, Accidental Suffocation or Strangulation in Bed does not have to occur in an actual bed, and may also occur when using a crib, couch, or armchair. This is why I prefer using the term SASS.

**Chaotic Bedsharing:** Sharing a bed or other sleep surface with an infant due to necessity rather than as an intentional parenting choice. Multiple hazardous risk factors are often present, such as other children or pets in the bed, parents being impaired by alcohol, drugs, or extreme exhaustion, one or more parent being a smoker, or a general lack of proactive sleep safety measures.

**Elective Bedsharing:** Sharing a bed with an infant as an intentional parenting and lifestyle choice, most often to facilitate breastfeeding or gain more sleep. Characterized by knowledge and avoidance of risk factors, and the parent's active and continuous commitment to the baby's safety.

**Mixed-Feeding:** Providing a baby with a combination of formula and breastmilk. Can include feeding the infant expressed breastmilk from a bottle, breastmilk directly from the breast, donor milk, and any variation of formula, cow's milk, or other milk substitute.

APPENDIX II

# Cosleeping Products

*Families who feel they are unable to maintain a safe bedsharing environment may use various products to create a separate-surface cosleeping arrangement that works for their unique family. Many parents may not be aware of what products are available and where they can find these devices, so the following is a list of suggested products designed to facilitate cosleeping. I am not recieving compensation for including any of these products in the book.*

## Arm's Reach® Versatile™ Co-Sleeper® Bedside Bassinet

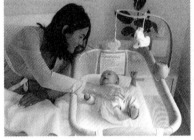

"The Versatile™ fits all types of beds. The adjustable feet can extend all the way under the bed allowing the bassinet to sit on top of your mattress. The feet are also retractable, allowing the bassinet to fit close to a platform bed or an adult bed that sits on the floor."

## Arm's Reach® Cambria Co-Sleeper® Bedside Bassinet

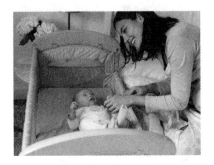

"This bedside bassinet features beautifully curved wooden ends, adjustable built-in leg extensions, and patented attachment strap and plate to provide the safest sleep solution."

## Arm's Reach® Co-Sleeper® Mini Ezee™ 2-in-1

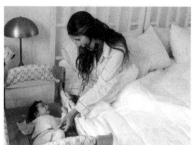

"The Co-Sleeper® Mini Ezee™ 2-in-1 is a safe way to bond with your infant as soon as they come home for the first time. It has more ventilation for even better breathability, side pockets and bottom compartment for storage, a 4-inch sleeping nest height, and an attachment strap and resistant plate."

## Baby Delight® Snuggle Nest® Harmony™ Infant Sleeper

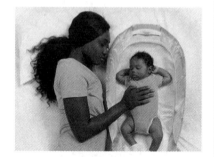

"Two rigid, vented wall units separate baby and your adult bedding while helping to prevent rollover. The sleeper's side panels are flexible, so it's simple to reach in and access your little one, and it features structural mesh for air circulation. A Sound & Light unit offers a gentle night light and soothing sounds of the womb or Brahms' Lullaby. The five-level volume control and automatic shut-off make it easy to adjust your young one's sleeping environment. When it's time for travel, the sleeper folds easily and compactly."

## The babybay® Bedside Bassinet

"Babybay®'s are half-moon shaped to mimic the protective feel of a hug. Solidly built, eco-friendly beechwood construction means your babybay® is strong, sustainable, durable, and made to last. Even if your baby outgrows the babybay® you can easily upgrade its size with a full-crib conversion kit. Customize your babybay® with a babynest®, adding softness, comfort, and style."

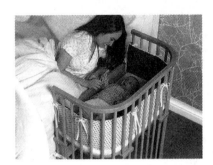

## HALO® Bassinest® Twin Sleeper

"The Halo® Bassinest® twin sleeper is the only space-saving bassinet for twins that rotates 360-degrees for the ultimate in convenience and safety. Now your little ones can sleep as close to you (and each other!) as you'd like, while still safely in their own separate sleep areas. Ideal for all moms of multiples, but especially moms who've had c-sections—as it makes it easy to tend to both babies without getting out of bed."

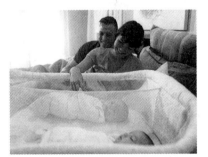

# APPENDIX III
# Cosleeping Resources and Further Reading

*These resources all pertain to safe infant sleep, but many of these contain conflicting information from institutions and entities that I critique, and whose interpretations and recommendations I disagree with when it comes to bedsharing and breastfeeding matters. Regardless of one's position on bedsharing, the more information made available, the better. Presenting all sides and persepctives allows for ideal decision-making. I think it's important that parents and professionals know what is being argued for, what is being argued against, and why.*

*Resources that fully match my personal recommendations are marked with the symbol appearing here:* ✔

## Books

✔ Berrozpe, María Martínez. *¡Dulces Sueños! (Sweet Sleep!)*. October, 2016. ISBN: 978-8441538368

> This book aspires to give a global, multidisciplinary, and integrative image of the science of children's sleep, and addresses parents' concerns about sleep problems.

Fleiss, Paul M. *Sweet Dreams: A Pediatrician's Secrets for Your Child's Good Night's Sleep*. December, 2000. ISBN: 978-0737304947

> Dr. Fleiss, a noted family pediatrician for more than 30 years, shares his secrets for discovering a child's natural sleep patterns, developing positive bedtime rituals, nutritional and lifestyle aids to sleep, and how cosleeping affects normal growth and development.

✔ Goodavage, Maria and Jay Gordon. *Good Nights: The Happy Parents' Guide to the Family Bed*. June, 2002. ISBN: 978-0312275181

> *Good Nights* puts your concerns about the family bed to rest, with fun and easy-to-use guidance on safety, coping with criticism, and even keeping the spark in your marriage (albeit outside the bedroom).

Jackson, Deborah. *Three in a Bed: The Benefits of Sharing Your Bed with Your Baby.* July, 2003. ISBN: 978-1582340517

> This classic book details the invaluable benefits of bedsharing for breastfeeding mothers, reviews the history of babies in the bed, and, through interviews with parents, explores current attitudes toward the idea.

✅ Kendall-Tackett, Kathleen and Wendy Middlemiss. *The Science of Mother-Infant Sleep.* October, 2013. ISBN: 978-1939807045

> A compilation of recent articles by an international group of experts on mother-baby sleep. It clarifies that parents must nurture children in order to allow the children to grow and develop normally; it also points out that there is no catch-all rulebook that parents can use to raise every child because each child has different needs. This text offers solutions for parents dealing with fatigue and ways to soothe a distressed baby.

✅ Michels, Dia L., Cyntia Good Mohab, and Naomi Bromberg Bar-Yam. *Breastfeeding at a Glance: Facts, Figures and Trivia About Lactation.* June, 2001. ISBN: 978-1930775053

> This comprehensive booklet answers frequently asked questions about breastfeeding, lists benefits for the family, and provides information on breastfeeding and the law, a resource list, and more.

Mindell, Jodi. *Sleeping Through the Night: How Infants, Toddlers, and Their Parents Can Get a Good Night's Sleep.* March, 2005. ISBN: 978-0060742560

> Mindell has ten years of experience in assessing and treating common sleep problems in children and uses her expertise in her book to provide parents with tips, answers to common questions, and quotes from parents who have solved their child's sleep problems.

✅ Mohrbacher, Nancy, and Kathleen Kendall-Tackett. *Breastfeeding Made Simple: Seven Natural Laws for Nursing Mothers.* 2005. ISBN: 978-1572248618

> This text informs parents of the benefits of breastfeeding, as well as cosleeping and other parenting techniques that increase the bond between child and parent.

Pantley, Elizabeth. *The No-Cry Sleep Solution.* March, 2002. ISBN: 978-0071381390

> Pantley provides solutions for how to get your baby to sleep at night with helpful strategies for overcoming naptime and bedtime problems with no crying and good nights of sleep.

✔ Sears, Martha, William Sears, and James Sears. *How to Get Your Baby to Sleep.* July, 2002. ISBN: 978-0316107716

> Dr. Bill and Martha Sears share their expertise on developing a nighttime routine, helping your child unwind at bedtime, the benefits of sleep-sharing, coping with a light sleeper or an early riser, and tips for getting your toddler to stay in bed.

✔ Sears, William. *Nighttime Parenting: How to Get your Baby and Child to Sleep.* November, 1999. ISBN: 978-0452281486

> Written to help the whole family sleep better, this book helps parents understand why babies sleep differently than adults and offers solutions to nighttime problems.

✔ Small, Meredith F. *Kids: How Biology and Culture Shape the Way We Raise Young Children.* October, 2002. ISBN: 978-0385496285

> Dr. Small discusses the development of preschool children aged one to six and offers new insights on deep-seated notions that are prescribed in many parenting books. She combines scientific research on human evolution and biology with her own observations of various cultures.

Sunderland, Margot. *Science of Parenting: Practical Guidance on Sleep, Crying, Play and Building Emotional Wellbeing for Life.* May, 2006. ISBN: 978-1405314862

> Based on over 700 scientific studies into children's development, child psychotherapist Dr. Margot Sunderland explains a hands-on parenting approach that helps children to realize their full potential.

Thevenin, Tine. *Family Bed.* February, 2002. ISBN: 978-0895293572

> An "excellent" (Jane Goodall, Ph.D.) guide to the pros and cons of having children sleep in their parents' beds. This book provides reassurance for parents who feel guilty about letting their children climb into bed with them.

Ockwell-Smith, Sarah. *Gentle Sleep Book.* March, 2015. ISBN: 978-0349405209

> This text offers gentle solutions to caring for children under five years old, including cosleeping in response to sleep inhibitors. Extensive scientific and anecdotal information helps the whole family get a good night's sleep.

Oster, Emily. *Cribsheet: A Data-Driven Guide to Better, More Relaxing Parenting, from Birth to Preschool.* April, 2019. ISBN: 978-0525559252

> Oster provides counterarguments to cosleeping recommendation, but emphasizes that the circumstances and personal choice of any parent can be the deciding factor on what the correct decision is for the individual.

Waldburger, Jennifer and Jill Spivack. *The Sleepeasy Solution: The Exhausted Parent's Guide to Getting Your Child to Sleep from Birth to Age 5.* April, 2007. ISBN: 978-0553394801

> From two experts who help the babies of Hollywood sleep, *The Sleepeasy Solution* provides a family-friendly guide to get children on a customized sleep schedule and addresses solutions to sleep problems.

Weissbluth, Marc. *Healthy Sleep Habits, Happy Child.* October, 2005. ISBN: 978-1511361453

> Dr. Weissbluth gives a step-by-step plan for parents to establish a sleep schedule that works with their child's natural sleep cycles. His book also reveals common mistakes made by parents when trying to get children to sleep, helps parents cope with common sleep problems, and more.

✅ West, Diana, Diane Wiessinger, Linda J. Smith, and Teresa Pitman. *Sweet Sleep: Nighttime and Naptime Strategies for the Breastfeeding Family.* July 2014. ISBN: 978-0345518477

> Information on nights and naps for breastfeeding families. It has mother-wisdom, reassurance, and a how-to guide for making safe decisions on how and where your family sleeps, backed by the latest research.

## Articles/Documents

American Academy of Pediatrics Report on SIDS.

> This 11-page report includes research on bedding, bedsharing, sleep position, pacifiers, immunizations, breastfeeding, and more in relation to SIDS and its prevention. Available at https://pediatrics.aappublications.org/content/pediatrics/138/5/e20162940.full.pdf

✅ Ball, Helen L. "Evolution-informed maternal-infant health." *Nature Ecology and Evolution, 1(3).* 2017.

> Dr. Ball demonstrates the tension in the mother-infant relationship by the contrast of the mother's ability to provide for the child to the neediness of the highly dependent human infant. Available at http://dro.dur.ac.uk/21367/1/21367.pdf?DDC89+DDD5+dan0hlb+d700tmt

✅ Ball, Helen L., Cecilia Tomori, and James J. McKenna. "Toward an Integrated Anthropology of Infant Sleep." *American Anthropologist, 121(3).* 2019.

> This article provides evidence that cosleeping combined with lactation represents a complex set of adaptations that constitute the human evolutionary norm. Available at https://doi.org/10.1111/aman.13284

✅ Bartick, Melissa and Cecilia Tomori. "Sudden infant death and social justice: A syndemics approach." *Maternal and Child Nutrition, 15.* 2019.

Report on physiological SIDS risk factors for infants. Available at https://onlinelibrary.wiley.com/doi/pdf/10.1111/mcn.12652

✅ Blunden, Sarah L., Kirrilly R. Thompson, and Drew Dawson. "Behavioural sleep treatments and night time crying in infants: challenging the status quo." *Sleep Medicine Review, 15(5).* 2011.

This paper debates whether an infant's cries should be ignored and ways in which sleep training techniques do or do not satisfy the needs of infants and parents. Available at https://doi.org/10.1016/j.smrv.2010.11.002

"Caring For Your Baby At Night: A Parent's Guide." UNICEF U.K., Baby Friendly Initiative, and Lullaby Trust. 2019.

This pamphlet is a thorough, eye-catching guide for bedsharing that covers everything from how to detect when your baby is ready for bedtime to the many rules for safe bedsharing. Available at https://www.unicef.org.uk/babyfriendly/baby-friendly-resources/sleep-and-night-time-resources/caring-for-your-baby-at-night/

✅ Gettler, Lee T. and James J. McKenna. "Never Sleep With Baby? Or Keep Me Close But Keep Me Safe: The Importance of Creating Appropriate Cosleeping Public Health Messages." *Current Pediatric Reviews, 6.* 2010.

This article details the reasons why it is necessary to provide the public with vital information on cosleeping. In order to promote safe cosleeping practices, parents must be informed enough to make the right decision for their family. Available at https://doi.org/10.2174/157339610791317250

✅ Marinelli, Kathleen A., Helen L. Ball, James J. McKenna, and Peter S. Blair. "An Integrated Analysis of Maternal-Infant Sleep, Breastfeeding, and Sudden Infant Death Syndrome Research Supporting a Balanced Discourse." *Journal of Human Lactation, 35(3).* 2019.

This analysis aims to review cosleeping and breastfeeding research through various lenses, and postulates the direction of future research to improve our knowledge and inform healthcare policy and practice. Available at https://doi.org/10.1177/0890334419851797

✅ McKenna, James J. and Lee T. Gettler. "There is no such thing as infant sleep, there is no such thing as breastfeeding, there is only breastsleeping." *Acta Paediatrica, 105(1),* 17–21. 2016.

This article is the first published work to define and describe the significance of the term "breastsleeping." Available at https://doi.org/10.1111/apa.13161

✅ McKenna, James J., Helen L. Ball, and Lee T. Gettler. "Mother-Infant Cosleeping, Breastfeeding and Sudden Infant Death Syndrome: What Biological Anthropology Has Discovered About Normal Infant Sleep and Pediatric Sleep Medicine." *Yearbook of Physical Anthropology, 50.* 2007.

This article delves deeper into understanding the connection between infant sleep patterns and medicine. It shows how science has come to better understand SIDS in recent years. Available at https://doi. org/10.1002/ajpa.20736

Riegle, Adrienne. "Ambivalence: New Research on Co-Sleeping in the United States." National Council on Family Relations. June, 2017.

The National Council on Family Relations (NCFR) and Dr. Riegle reduce the stigma of cosleeping while informing parents of the psychological advantages. Available at https://www.ncfr.org/ncfr-report/focus/ ambivalence-new-research-co-sleeping-united-states

✅ "SIDS: The Latest Research on How Sleeping With Your Baby is Safe." Ask Dr. Sears: A Trusted Resource for Parents.

This is an informative article that describes the history of sleeping with babies and lists the dos and don'ts when sharing a bed with your baby. Available at: http://www.askdrsears.com/html/10/t102200.asp

"Sleeping with Your Baby—Cosleeping Issue I," *Mothering Magazine Special Edition*, September/October 2002.

This 40-page reprint from *Mothering Magazine* provides research to support cosleeping, as well as practical information and safety guidelines. Available at http://www.motheringshop.com/

Wiessinger, Diane, Diana West, Linda J. Smith, and Teresa Pitman. "The Safe Sleep Seven." La Leche League International. 2018.

This article discusses contrasting theories regarding infant sleep and breastfeeding by weighing the pros and cons of both sides of the argument. Available at https://www.llli.org/the-safe-sleep-seven/

✅ "Who Wants to Sleep Alone—Cosleeping Issue II," *Mothering Magazine Special Edition*, January/February 2009.

This reprint features two helpful articles: "The Science of Sharing Sleep" by Lee T. Gettler and James J. McKenna and "The Solace of the Family Bed" by Sarah J. Buckley, M.D. It also includes 48 inspiring cosleeping photos. Available at http://www.motheringshop.com/

# Instructor Resources

✅ Baby Sleep Info Source (Basis). Outreach arm of the Durham Infancy & Sleep Centre (DISC).

> The aim of Basis is to provide online access to up-to-date research about infant sleep, in forms that are accessible to parents and health practitioners. The website offers infant sleep education workshops for professionals, information sheets, leaflets, key resarch summaries, the Infant Sleep Info app, and other resources. Available at http://www.BasisOnline.org.uk

"Health Professional's Guide to Caring For Your Baby At Night." UNICEF UK, Baby Friendly Initiative, and the Foundation for the Study of Infant Deaths. 2017.

> This pamphlet is a thorough, eye-catching guide for bedsharing that covers everything from how to detect when your baby is ready for bedtime to the many rules for safe bedsharing. Available at https://www.unicef.org.uk/babyfriendly/baby-friendly-resources/sleep-and-night-time-resources/caring-for-your-baby-at-night/

✅ McKenna, James J. *Sleep Like a Baby* PowerPoint presentation slides.

> Dr. McKenna uses these presentations to inform people of the benefits of cosleeping, who opposes it and why, and what evidence there is on both sides of the argument. Available at https://cosleeping.nd.edu/assets/56157/sleep_like_a_baby.pdf

# DVDs/Videos

*7 Steps To Reduce The Risk of SIDS*. Childbirth Graphics. 2006.

> Based on information from the AAP, this DVD shows viewers how to lower the risk of SIDS through simple safety steps. It can be purchased in English or Spanish. Available at http://www.childbirthgraphics.com

✅ *Fatal Mistake*. A Fox 6 Investigative Report on cosleeping deaths in Milwaukee.

> Watch this compelling investigative report explore what a number of SIDS deaths in Milwaukee between 2010–2012 had in common. Featuring interviews with Dr. James J. McKenna, this video is a must-see for maternal and child health professionals and parents alike! Available at http://platypusmedia.com/safe-sleep

Gilbert, Paul and Wendi. *Sleep Like a Baby*, Professional edition (includes viewing rights in professional/educational settings and free access to an online resource folder). 2010.

> By providing a thorough overview of the topic, debunking myths, and helping set realistic expectations, this educational DVD enables parents to make safe sleep choices. Professional and Home editions available at http://sleepbaby.com/store.html

Goldmacher, Donald and Michael Fox. *Helping Your Baby Sleep Through the Night*. 2006.

> This DVD offers step-by-step sleep hygiene advice to allow parents and their child to have restful nights of sleep. Their advice is based on research done at Stanford University Infant Sleep Laboratory as well as from other child experts. Available at http://helpingyourbabysleep.com/index.php

Spivock, Jill and Jennifer Waldburger. *The Sleepeasy Solution: The Complete Guide to Getting Your Baby or Toddler to Sleep*. 2007.

> The authors of *The Sleepeasy Solution* book have created this DVD based on their book. The DVD leads parents step-by-step to solve their baby's sleeping problems and provide footage of real families solving sleep problems. Available at http://www.sleepyplanet.com

✔ McKenna, James J. Videos and interviews.

> Watch Dr. McKenna as he informs, educates, reassures, and defends cosleeping in an array of news investigations, documentaries, and university productions. Available at www.cosleeping.nd.edu/videos/

## Product Reviews

Consumer Reports: Baby Products.

> Consumer Reports has a whole section of their website dedicated to babies and kids. Ratings can be found for nearly all baby products from car seats to bottles. Available at http://www.consumerreports.org/cro/babies-kids/index.htm

Consumer Product Safety Commission: Crib Safety and SIDS Reduction Information.

> This website includes publications, brochures, and safety alerts about crib safety and safe sleeping. Available at https://www.cpsc.gov/Safety-Education/Safety-Education-Centers/cribs

# Organizations

✅ **The Academy of Breastfeeding Medicine** is a worldwide organization of physicians dedicated to the promotion, protection, and support of human breastfeeding and lactation.

Visit www.bfmed.org

**The American Academy of Pediatrics (AAP)** dedicates their efforts and resources to the health, safety, and well-being of infants, children, adolescents, and young adults.

Visit www.pediatrics.aappublications.org

**The Association of Maternal and Child Health Programs (AMCHP)** is a national resource, partner, and advocate for state public health leaders and others working to improve the health of women, children, youth, and families, including those with special health care needs.

Visit www.amchp.org

✅ **Attachment Parenting International (API)**, in addition to helping form Attachment Parenting support groups, functions as a clearinghouse providing educational materials, research information, consultative, referral, and speaker services to promote Attachment Parenting concepts.

Visit www.attachmentparenting.org

**Baby Sleep Information Source** is a project of the Durham University Parent-Infant Sleep Lab. It offers infant sleep training workshops and provides safe infant sleep information sheets, a safe sleep app, and other resources.

Visit www.basisonline.org.uk

✅ **The Durham Infancy & Sleep Centre (DISC)** is a research centre, run by Dr. Helen L. Ball, studying infancy and sleep, based in the Department of Anthropology at Durham University, U.K. Formerly the Parent-Infant Sleep Lab.

Visit www.dur.ac.uk/disc

**First Candle** provides information for new and expectant parents guiding them from pregnancy to the baby's first birthday, as well as information for grieving parents. Their "Safe Sleep Saves Lives" pamphlet provides a well-informed list of safe sleep rules to protect your baby from SIDS and accidents while room sharing.

Visit www.firstcandle.org

**Global Infant Safe Sleep Center (GISS)** supports vulnerable and marginalized global communities in an effort to reduce Sudden Unexpected Infant Death. Their mission is to empower the world's communities by achieving equity in infant survival.

Visit www.gisscenter.org

**Healthy Child Care America** (a program of the American Academy of Pediatrics) addresses both general and specific guidelines concerning pediatric issues by providing information on the AAP's programs, policies, guidelines, publications, and more. The website provides a flyer, "A Parent's Guide to Safe Sleep: Helping you to reduce the risk of SIDS," which informs parents about SIDS and about how to sleep near your baby safely.

Visit www.healthychildcare.org

**Healthy Children** is the only parenting website backed by 60,000 pediatricians committed to the attainment of optimal physical, mental, and social health and well-being for all infants, children, adolescents, and young adults.

Visit www.healthychildren.org

**International Society for the Study and Prevention of Perinatal and Infant Death (ISPID)** is a non-profit organization geared towards research to prevent stillbirth and infant death as well as promoting improved care for affected parents.

Visit www.ispid.org

✓ **La Leche League International** is a mother-to-mother support group whose mission is to help mothers worldwide to breastfeed through mother-to-mother support, education, information, and encouragement and to promote a better understanding of breastfeeding as an important element in the healthy development of the baby and mother.

Visit www.llli.org

**The Lullaby Trust** is a British charitable organization aiming to prevent unexpected deaths in infancy and promote infant health.

Visit www.lullabytrust.org.uk

**March of Dimes** is a non-profit organization aimed at improving the health of babies by preventing premature births, birth defects, and infant mortality through education, advocacy, research, and community services.

Visit www.marchofdimes.com

⊘ **The Mother-Baby Behavioral Sleep Lab** is based in the Department of Anthropology at the University of Notre Dame, previously directed by Dr. James J. McKenna. The lab studies how sleeping environments reflect and respond to family needs—in particular how they affect mothers, breastfeeding, and infants' physiological and psychological well-being and development.

Visit www.cosleeping.nd.edu/

**National Action Partnership to Promote Safe Sleep (NAPPSS)** is an initiative to make infant safe sleep and breastfeeding the national norm.

Visit www.nichq.org

**National Institute of Child Health and Human Development (NICHD)** conducts and supports research on all stages of human development, from preconception to adulthood, to better understand the health of children, adults, families, and communities.

Visit www.nichd.nih.gov

**National Sudden and Unexpected Infant/Child Death & Pregnancy Loss Resource Center (NSIDRC)** is a central source of information on sudden infant death and works to promote healthy outcomes for infants through the first year of life and beyond. The website includes a list of pertinent topics from A to Z, including a section on safe sleep.

Visit www.sidscenter.org

**U.S. Consumer Product Safety Commission (CPSC)** has the task of ensuring the public's safety against serious injury or death from thousands of types of consumer products. Their website features a section entitled Crib Information Center, which offers information about recalled cribs as well as resources pertaining to crib safety.

Visit www.cpsc.gov

**Zero to Three** is a national, nonprofit organization that informs, trains, and supports professionals, policymakers, and parents in their efforts to improve the lives of infants and toddlers.

Visit www.zerotothree.org

APPENDIX IV

# Cosleeping Saves Lives:
## First-Hand Accounts
## From Real Parents

*The following pages contain real descriptions from families about what cosleeping means to them and how it has helped their infants stay safe and healthy throughout the night. These responses were recorded in 2007 in "An Internet Based Study of Infant Sleeping Arrangements and Parental Perceptions."[36] All submissions were anonymous to protect the privacy of the survey partipants. Quotes were edited for clarity and style.*

### Account 1

When our fifth child was born, we again coslept and nursed. When she was just six weeks old, I suddenly awoke one night because I felt that something was wrong. I reached over and touched her, and she wasn't breathing and was cold to the touch. I screamed and started shaking her, and she took a deep breath and started to breathe. We took her to the doctor, who found nothing wrong and said I must have been dreaming. Two days later, I had placed her in the bassinet next to my bed after she had fallen asleep nursing. I felt the impulse a short time later to check on her. Once again, she was not breathing and was turning blue. I grabbed her and dropped her on my bed, screaming, and once again she took a deep breath and started breathing.

After running tests, the doctors found that she was sleeping too deeply at times and forgetting to breathe. They hooked her to a monitor, and between the monitor and having her with me both during the day in a body carrier and at night in bed, she made it through her first year until her brain reached a maturity that it remembered to breathe even when she was sleeping. I had one doctor tell me that if I had not been so in tune with my baby—being awakened by her the first time, and checking on her the second—she probably would have been a SIDS baby.

## Account 2

We have had a family bed for all three children with great outcomes. Once when my second daughter was six months old, I woke up suddenly because she stopped breathing. There was nothing obstructing her face, no pillows, blankets, people, or anything, and I reached over to touch her chest, which was not moving. I picked her up and gently shook her four times before she gasped loudly and started breathing again. I was scared I hurt her when I shook her, but I didn't do it very hard. I hate to think what could have happened if she had been in a crib and I did not notice her sudden silence. I spoke to her pediatrician about this the next morning. It happened again when she was nine months old, the same exact way, except I rocked her back and forth as her doctor suggested instead of shaking her. She also has a seizure history, and I have woken up at least once, maybe twice, when she was having a seizure next to me. She is three and a half now and still sleeps with us most nights.

My oldest used to spike high fevers (up to 106 °F) in the night. She would not cry out or anything. I would notice when I touched her in my sleep and felt her burning up. Then I would know to get up and treat her.

## Account 3

I did not cosleep by design with my first child until he was about nine months old. My child had a short frenulum, which was diagnosed by his pediatrician and commented on by a nurse when he was newborn, but no one knew that this could give him trouble with breastfeeding. Since he was such an inefficient nurser, he had to be at the breast almost continuously day and night. This turned out to be a blessing because it ensured that I had to learn to bedshare with him, which in turn ensured all our babies reaped the benefits of cosleeping. Although I tried to do the typical American thing—get him to sleep in a crib—I was utterly unsuccessful at this and he never spent more than 10–20 minutes in it a night. I would nurse sitting up in bed (a bed on a frame, with a footboard and a headboard) trying to stay awake so I could put him back in the crib when he seemed asleep. This was exhausting. I once dropped him when I fell asleep sitting up, and he fell out of the bed onto the floor. After that episode I abandoned the idea of trying to stay awake while nursing…I took my bed apart, put the mattress on the floor, and began to nurse while lying on my side.

## Account 4

We bedshare with our two-year-old son. When he was five months old, one night I awoke to some moving and noticed my son was blue. There was NOTHING around him and he was on top of the blanket in a shirt, but was not breathing. I picked him up and gave him some thumps on his back and he started crying. We took him to the hospital and the doctor concluded he must have had a mucus plug. Had he been in his own bed, I would not have known and I would have lost him. From that day on we were FIRM believers in cosleeping....I pray to God that he let us keep him, and I am so thankful I had become "lazy" in my parenting and just left him in bed with me.

## Account 5

When our older boy was about six weeks old, I woke to find him choking next to me. He was on his back, had spit up, and could not clear his mouth. He didn't make a sound—I don't know what woke me. I rolled him on his side, the spit-up came out, and he was fine. I honestly don't know if he could have cleared it himself or not. I DO know that, had he been in another room, I would not have woken up to help him.

## Account 6

Throughout his first year of life, our five-year-old son (for no reason we knew of) would just stop breathing. When we would rouse him, he would then gasp for air. He now has serious asthma. We think, and the doctor agrees, that this was possibly a pre-asthma situation he was going through. I believe without such careful monitoring and the constant motion of people around him in bed, we could have had serious consequences.

## Account 7

My daughter, at age two months, was sleeping propped up because of gastroesophageal reflux. She once fell off the little mattress we were using to prop her up with, and was hanging off it, face down. I immediately woke up (interestingly, because I had a dream where my son told me to wake up because she was in danger) and was able to place her on her back.

## Account 8

Our baby had difficulties breathing for the first couple of days, with minor apneas and rushed breathing and some tachycardia. But over the course of a few days, that seemed to resolve itself. He was a very weak and sleepy baby.

He slept with me from the first night home. I made a little elevated baby nest for him as he had a bit of reflux. On the second night home I woke up to find he had a pause in his breathing. I felt a bit panicked and rubbed his chest, and he started to breathe immediately upon touching him. I thought it must have been my imagination.

When my baby was three months old, my nightmare began. I had nursed him to sleep after a night of much fussing and crying. He had been a really happy and contented baby until about two weeks before, when he received his DPT. From that day he started a pattern where he would cry for hours at a time with nothing to soothe him. He sounded like he was hurting. It didn't seem like colic (which my firstborn had).

That night after I had nursed him to sleep in my bed, I fell asleep myself. At about three in the morning, I awoke with my senses just screaming "LOOK AT THE BABY!" I looked over to where he lay in the bed and he just glowed this horrible white color. It was awful. He was so still. His chest was not moving. I leaned over him to feel for his breath on my face, but there was none. I put my hand on his chest; it was not moving. I rubbed my hand on his chest, jiggling him a bit. Panic set in at this point. I did it again, only this time more rigorously. All of a sudden he took this ghastly breath in that was so forceful it lurched his tiny chest up in the air a bit. It was so deep and sudden, it was like he was sucking the life back into him.

I woke him up, cried my eyes out, and put him to the breast. I was told by his doctor that it was apnea. He consulted with a specialist. It was determined that there was nothing that we could do. We could have used a monitor, but they felt that that would disrupt our family too much. I slept fitfully for weeks with my baby on my chest, hoping that my heartbeat and the sound of my breathing would remind him to keep going.

Eventually he didn't want to sleep on me anymore. We built a cosleeper and bought an angel-care monitor to track his breathing. That just made us crazy, and nobody slept well. The foot of space between us seemed as wide as an ocean. He moved back to his space beside me, and there he has slept ever since. He is now 20 months old, strong and vibrant. Happy as can be, and the joy of our family.

## Account 9

At one point, both my twins had colds (they were about three months old) and had difficulty breathing. We used physiological solution to purge their noses and had drops given to us by the doctor, but not much was working. All of a sudden one night, my husband and I woke up with a jump at the same moment: One of our daughters had made the smallest little sound—just an "urp"—that alarmed us both out of sleep. We immediately turned on the light and there she was, turning red-blue. She couldn't breathe. We purged her nose and then my husband took her downstairs to the bathroom where he ran a hot shower and sat with her in the steamy room. He came back ten minutes later and she was breathing freely.

We're both certain that if she'd been in another room, or even in another bed, we would NOT have heard the little sound she made. Having her right beside us alerted us to the change in her breathing, even though we were sleeping.

Also, my husband is convinced that he's much more attached to his girls as a result of sleeping with them: Waking up to three smiling faces every morning that are happy as can be to see him has made him feel... great.

## Account 10

Cosleeping definitely saved my son's life. I am now a La Leche League Leader in the U.K., and I am the first to suggest safe cosleeping to mothers. My son was a colicky baby for three months, and he cried all day and all night. During the day he was carried around in a sling, and if we napped it was in the family bed (a double sprung mattress with sheets and covers). At night we either walked the floors in the bedroom, laid on the bed to breastfeed, or dozed off on the bed after a feed. When the colic subsided we continued to sleep together in the double bed. At four months of age, he was ill during the day. He had a temperature and was sleepy (very unusual for him). We gave him Calpol (paediatric paracetamol) but we weren't unduly worried until he started to refuse breastfeeds at night, and his breathing became irregular. We called a doctor but he told us the baby had an ear infection and we should continue giving him Calpol. Having slept with my son for four months I knew him so well—the touch of his skin told me he was very hot, his breathing wasn't in its normal pattern, he refused the breast, his gaze seemed distant. I demanded that a different doctor come out to our house. His prognosis was the same as the last doctor's, and made it seem like we were unduly worrying.

By the morning I was frantic with worry. My son was dehydrated from refusing feeds all night, and was making whimpering noises that I hadn't heard before. He didn't seem like MY BABY at all, nor did his skin SMELL the same to me. A third doctor came at 10 AM that morning and decided to send us to the local hospital because of the dehydration. At the Accident and Emergency Unit a doctor examined him in detail and then went to seek a Consultant. The Consultant told us that our son had suspected Meningitis, and we were rushed to a quarantine room for an immediate lumbar puncture to be done on him. The results came back that afternoon and we were given the bad news that he had Pneumococcal Meningitis and it had not been caught in its early stages! To this day I believe that if the doctors had listened to my reports and I had been taken seriously, we would have caught the infection in its early stages instead. Our son did recover. I gave him my expressed breastmilk and as he became more alert, I breastfed him over the sides of his cot. The Consultant Paediatrician said that my breastmilk had helped in his recovery. I am now a firm supporter of cosleeping, as long as safety rules are followed to ensure there is no risk of entrapment. My husband and I also do not drink. You really get to know your infant well when you breastfeed and cosleep—so much so it just might save a life!

## Account 11

Our daughter had obvious cessations of breathing and would choke numerous times while sleeping and upon awakening. It was quite frightening, and happened even until the age of sleeping upright in an infant car seat. This choking never happened while awake. It was also worse when she was lying flat on her back, so I often slept half upright against a bed pillow with her on my chest, tummy to tummy. This kept her airway clear. Being prone at a 45 degree angle seemed the best for her, especially when teething, because she had a lot of mucous during that time, accompanied by a feverish state with each tooth. At age 21, she had the same symptoms with four impacted wisdom teeth attempting to erupt. She had them surgically removed and symptoms disappeared.

## Account 12

I believe our youngest would not be alive today had she slept out of our sight. She was a foster child placed with us at birth. Diagnosed IUGR (born small but carried full term), she thrived for eight weeks. She then developed an occasional cough; the cough itself was frightening, but it occurred only two or three times a day. She did not have a fever or other symptoms, and she looked and behaved normally between coughing spells. I slept with her propped up on my chest the last two nights before she was hospitalized with pertussis (which took two days of outpatient testing to diagnose—testing that was done only because my pediatrician trusted my judgment that this was an atypical cough). I believe that, had she slept elsewhere, she would have quietly choked to death any night that week before diagnosis. So many parents of SIDS babies say, "She only had a little cough."

# APPENDIX V
# Anti-Bedsharing Campaigns

*Public health messages about the dangers of bedsharing tend to be intense, frightening, vilifying, judgmental, and focused on shock value. Yet, despite the hard-hitting imagery and bold slogans in the following examples, the campaigns have failed to stop the practice of bedsharing.*

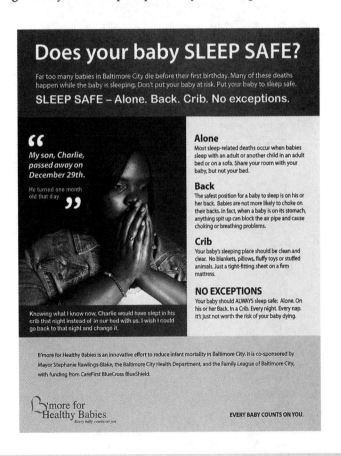

Baltimore City Health Department in partnership with the Family League of Baltimore. B'more for Healthy Babies. Sleep Safe Campaign. Baltimore, MD. 2013.

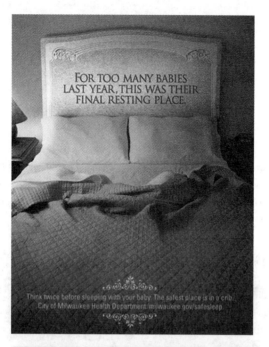

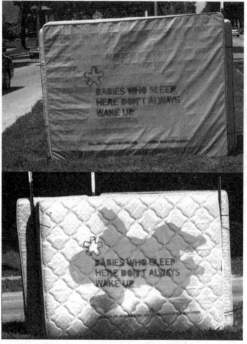

The Milwaukee Health Department. Safe Sleep Campaign.
Milwaukee, WI. January 2010–July 2012.

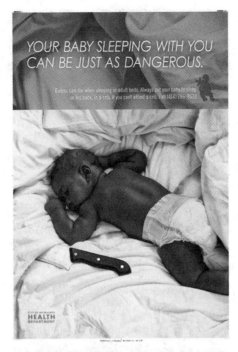

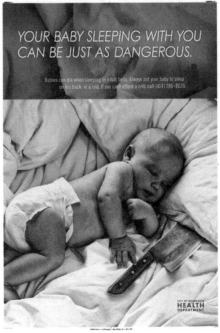

The Milwaukee Health Department. Safe Sleep Campaign.
Milwaukee, WI. January 2010–July 2012.

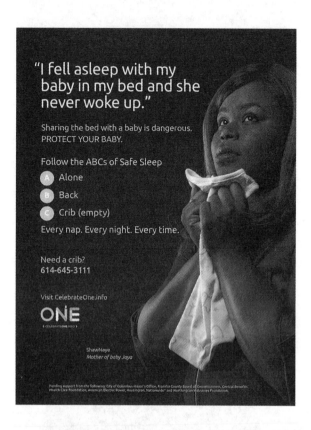

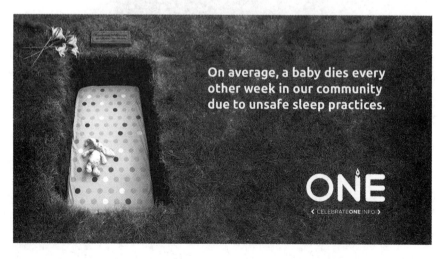

The City of Columbus. CelebrateOne. Safe Sleep Campaign.
Columbus, OH. 2015.

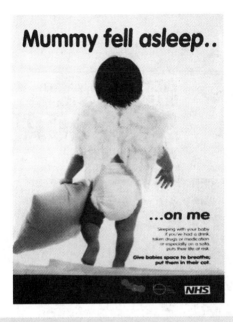

National Health Services. Safe Sleep Campaign.
Birmingham, England. 2012.

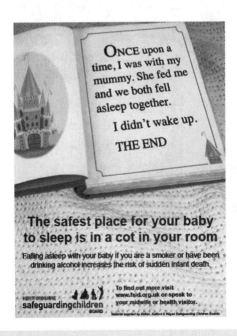

Hertfordshire Safeguarding Children Board. HSCB Safe Sleeping Campaign.
Hertfordshire County, England. April 2012.

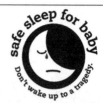

# EVERY 5 DAYS, A BABY IN LOS ANGELES COUNTY
# SUFFOCATES
## WHILE SLEEPING.

### IS YOUR BABY SLEEPING SAFELY?

Share a room, not a bed

Lay baby down to sleep in a crib or bassinet

Place babies on their back every time, at night and for naps

Give babies space to breathe — no pillows, bumpers, blankets or toys

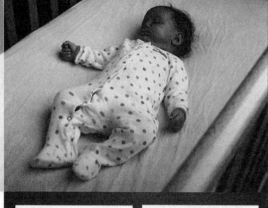

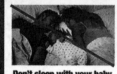

Don't sleep with your baby

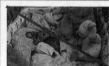

Don't let your baby sleep in a crowded crib

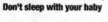

## DON'T WAKE UP TO A TRAGEDY

ICAN
ican4kids.org

first 5 la
Giving kids the best start

www.SafeSleepForBaby.com    info@safesleepforbaby.com

LA County Health Department. Safe Sleep For Baby.
LA County Infant Safe Sleeping Campaign. Los Angeles County, CA. 2019.

# APPENDIX VI
# List of Figures

# APPENDIX VII
# References

1. Marinelli, K.A., Ball, H.L., McKenna, J.J., & Blair, P.S. (2019). An Integrated Analysis of Maternal-Infant Sleep, Breastfeeding, and Sudden Infant Death Syndrome Research Supporting a Balanced Discourse. *Journal of Human Lactation, 35(3)*, 510–520. doi:10.1177/0890334419851797

2. McKenna, J.J. & Gettler, L.T. (2016). There is no such thing as infant sleep, there is no such thing as breastfeeding, there is only breastsleeping. *Acta Paediatrica, 105(1)*, 17–21.

3. McKenna, J.J. & Gettler, L.T. (2017). Supporting a Bottom-Up, New, No-Holds-Barred, Psych-Anthro-Pediatrics: Making Room (Scientifically) For Bedsharing Families. *Sleep Medicine Reviews.* doi:10.1016/j.smry.2016.06.003

4. Goldman, A.S. (2018). Future research in the immune system of human milk. *The Journal of Pediatrics.* doi:10.1016/j.peds.2018.11.024

5. Lester, B.M., Conrad, T.E., LaGasse, L.L., Tronick, E.Z., Padbury, J.F., & Marsit, C.J. (2018). Epigenetic Programming by Maternal Behavior in the Human Infant. *Pediatrics, 142(4).*

6. Winnicott, D.W. (1964). *The Child, the Family and the Outside World.* London: Penguin Books.

7. Hardyment, C. (1983). *Dream Babies: Childcare from Locke to Spock.* London: Jonathan Cape.

8. McKenna, J.J., Ball, H.L., & Gettler, L.T. (2007). Mother-infant cosleeping, breastfeeding and sudden infant death syndrome: What biological anthropology has discovered about normal infant sleep and pediatric sleep medicine. *American Journal of Physical Anthropology, 134(S45)*, 133–61. doi:10.1002/ajpa.20736

9. Rodrigues, M.A. & Clancy, B.H.K. (2017). Costly and Cute: Helpless Infants and Human Evolution. *American Journal of Human Biology: The official journal of the Human Biology Council, 29(4)*, 295–231. doi:10.1002/ajhb.23019. Wenda R. Trevathan and Karen R. Rosenberg (Eds.), NM: University of New Mexico Press.

10. McKenna, J.J. (2017). Mother-Infant Dyad. *International Encyclopedia of Biological Anthropology.* W.R. Trevathen. (Eds.) Wiley: New York.

11. McKenna, J.J., Mosko, S., Dungy, C., & McAninch, J. (1990). Sleep and Arousal Patterns of Co-Sleeping Human Mother-Infant Pairs: A Preliminary Physiological Study with Implications for the Study of the Sudden Infant Death Syndrome (SIDS). *American Journal of Physical Anthropology, 82(3)*, 331–347.

12. McKenna, J.J., Mosko, S., & Richard, C. (1997). Bedsharing promotes breastfeeding. *Pediatrics, 100*, 214–219.

13. McKenna, J.J., Mosko S., Richard, C., Drummond, S., Hunt, L., Cetal, M., & Arpaia, J. (1994). Mutual behavioral and physiological influences among solitary and co-sleeping mother-infant pairs; implications for SIDS. *Early Human Development, 38*, 182–201.

14. Baddock, S.A., Galland, B.C., Bolton, D.P.G, Williams, S., & Taylor, B.J. (2006). Differences in infant and parent behaviors during routine bed sharing compared with cot sleeping in the home setting. *The Journal of Pediatrics, 117*, 1599–1607.

15. Baddock, S.A., Galland, B.C., Taylor, B.J., & Bolton, D.P.G. (2007). Sleep arrangements and behavior of bed-sharing families in the home setting. *Pediatrics, 119*, e200–e207.

16. Ball, H.L. (2002). Reasons to bed-share: why parents sleep with their infants. *Journal of Reproductive and Infant Psychology, 20(4)*, 207–221.

17. Blair, P.S., et al. (2014). Bed-Sharing in the Absence of Hazardous Circumstances: Is There a Risk of Sudden Infant Death Syndrome? An Analysis from Two Case-Control Studies Conducted in the UK. *PLoS ONE, 9(9).* doi:10.1371/journal.pone.0107799

18. Parades, M.F., et al. (2016). Extensive migration of young neurons into the infant human frontal lobe. *Science, 354(6308).* doi:10.1126/science.aaf7073

19. Mosko, S., McKenna, J.J., et al. (1993). Infant-Parent Co-sleeping: The Appropriate Context for the Study of Infant Sleep and Implications for SIDS. *Journal of Behavioral Medicine, 16(6)*, 589–610.

20. Hahn, R. Personal communication.

21.  Hrdy, S.B. (2000). *Mother Nature: Maternal Instincts and How They Shape the Human Species*. New York: Ballantine Books.

22.  Montagu, A.T. (1986). *Touching: The Human Significance of the Skin*. (3rd edition). NY: Harper Row.

23.  Hrdy, S.B. (1999). *The Natural History of Mothers, Infants and Natural Selection*. NY: Pantheon.

24.  Field, T.M. (1998). Touch therapy effects on development. *International Journal of Behavioral Development, 22*, 779–797.

25.  Field, T.M., et al. (1986). Tactile/kinesthetic stimulation effects on preterm neonates. *The Journal of Pediatrics, 77*, 654–658.

26.  Murdock, G.P., Ford, C.S., Hudson, A.E., Kennedy, R., Simmons, L.W., & Whiting, J.W.M. (2006). *Outline of Cultural Materials (6th ed.)*. New Haven, CT: Human Relations Area Files.

27.  Whiting, J.W.M. (1981). Environmental constraints on infant care practices. *Handbook of Cross-Cultural Human Development*. R.H. Munroe, R.L. Munroe, and B.B. Whiting. (Eds.) NY: Garland STPM Press.

28.  Ball, H.L. & Klingaman, P.K. (2007). Breastfeeding and mother-infant sleep proximity: implications for infant care. *Evolutionary Medicine and Health: New Perspectives*. NY: Oxford University Press. 226–241.

29.  Flandrin, J.L. (1979). *Families in Former Times: Kinship, Household and Sexuality*. Translated by R. Southern. (Themes in the Social Sciences.) NY: Cambridge University Press.

30.  Kellum, B.A. (1974). Infanticide in England in the later Middle Ages. *History of Childhood Quarterly. Winter; 1(3)*, 367–88.

31.  Keller, M.A. & Goldberg, W.A. (2004). Co-sleeping: Help or hindrance for young children's independence? *Infant and Child Development, 13*, 369–388. doi:10.1002/icd.365

32.  Field, T.M. (2001). Massage therapy facilitates weight gain in preterm infants. *Current Directions in Psychological Science, 10*, 51–54.

33.  Mosko, S., Richard, C., & McKenna, J.J. (1997). Maternal sleep and arousals during bedsharing with infants. *Sleep, 20(2)*, 142–150.

34.  Nelson, E.A., et al. (2001). International Child Care Study: Infant Sleeping Environment. *Early Human Development, 62(1)*, 43–55.

35.  McKenna, J.J., Thoman, E.B., Anders, T.F., Sadeh, A., Schechtman, V.L., & Glotzbach, S.F. (1993). Infant-parent co-sleeping in an evolutionary perspective: implications for understanding infant sleep development and the sudden infant death syndrome. *Sleep, 16(3)*, 263–282.

36.  McKenna, J.J. & Volpe, L. (2007). An Internet Based Study of Infant Sleeping Arrangements and Parental Perceptions. Infant Behavior and Child Development special issue on cosleeping. Wendy Goldberg. (Ed.) *Infant and Child Development, 16*, 359–385. doi:10.1002/icd.525

37.  Kendall-Tackett, K., Cong, Z., & Hale, T.W. (2010). Mother-Infant Sleep Locations and Nighttime Feeding Behavior: U.S. Data from the Survey of Mothers' Sleep and Fatigue. *Clinical Lactation, 1(1)*, 27–31.

38.  Mitchell, E.A. (2009). SIDS: past, present and future. *Acta Pædiatrica, 98(11)*, 1712–1719. doi:10.1111/j.1651-2227.2009.01503.x

39.  Moon, R.Y. & Hauck, F.R. (2015). SIDS Risk: It's More Than Just the Sleep Environment. *Pediatrics, 137(1)*. doi:10.1542/peds.2015-3665.

40.  Freed, G. & Martinez, F. (2017). The History of Home Cardiorespiratory Monitoring. *Pediatric Annals, 46(8)*. doi:10.3928/19382359-20170725-01

41.  Strehle, E.M., et al. (2011). Can Home Monitoring Reduce Mortality in Infants at Increased Risk of Sudden Infant Death Syndrome? A Systematic Review. *Acta Paediatrica, 101(1)*, 8–13. doi:10.1111/j.1651-2227.2011.02464.x

42.  Moon, R.Y. (2011). From the American Academy of Pediatrics Policy Statement. SIDS and Other Sleep-Related Infant Deaths: Expansion of Recommendations for a Safe Infant Sleeping Environment. *Pediatrics, 128(5)*, 1030–1039. doi:10.1542/peds.2011-2284

43.  Hicks, C. (2011). The Truth about Baby Breathing Monitors. *The Independent*. Independent Digital News and Media. Retrieved from www.independent.co.uk/life-style/health-and-families/health-news/the-truth-about-baby-breathing-monitors-1251950.html

44. Liu, G., et al. (2015). Home Apnea Monitors—When to Discontinue Use. *The Journal of Family Practice, 64(12),* 769–772. Retrieved from https://www.mdedge. com/sites/default/files/issues/articles/media_8fd2fa1_JFP_06412_Article1.PDF

45. Barry, E. (2017). Why Rates of Bedsharing With Infants Are Rising, While U.S. Health Policy Advocates Condemn It. *National Council on Family Relations.* Retrieved from www.ncfr.org/ncfr-report/focus/why-rates-bedsharing-infants-are-rising

46. Hauck, F.R., Herman, S.M., Donovan, M., et al. (2003). Sleep environment and the risk of Sudden Infant Death Syndrome in an urban population: the Chicago Infant Mortality Study. *Pediatrics, 111(5),* 1207–1214.

47. Baddock, S.A., Purnell, M.T., Blair, P.S., Pease, A., Elder, D., & Galland, B. (2019). The influence of bedsharing on infant physiology, breastfeeding and behavior: a systematic review. *Sleep Medicine Review, 43,* 106–117.

48. McKenna, J.J. (2002). Breastfeeding and Bedsharing: Still Useful (and Important) After All These Years. *Mothering Magazine, 114,* 28–37.

49. Erck Lambert, A.B., Parks, S.E., Cottengim, C., Faulkner, M., Hauck, F.R., Shapiro-Mendoza, C.K. (2019). Sleep-Related Infant Suffocation Deaths Attributable to Soft Bedding, Overlay, and Wedging. *Pediatrics, 143(5).* doi:10.1542/peds.2018-3408

50. Blair, P.S., personal communication, March 19, 2019.

51. Ball, H.L. (2017). The Atlantic Divide: Contrasting U.K. and U.S. Recommendations on Cosleeping and Bed-sharing. *Journal of Human Lactation,* 1–5.

52. Côté, A. (2006). Bed sharing and sudden infant death syndrome: Do we have a definition problem? *Paediatrics and Child Health, 11 (Suppl. LA),* 34–38. doi:10.1093/pch/11.supple_A.34A

53. Actman, H.B. (2016). Are You Among the 46 Percent of Parents Who Lie About This? A poll reveals a surprising number of parents lie about co-sleeping with their kids. *Parenting Magazine.* Retrieved from www.parents.com/baby/all-about-babies/are-you-among-the-46-percent-of-parents-who-lie-about-this/

54. Ball, H.L., Hooker, E., & Kelly, P.J. (1999). Where will the baby sleep? Attitudes and practices of new and experienced parents regarding cosleeping with their newborn infants. *American Anthropologist, 101(1),* 143–151.

55. Blair, P.S., Sidebotham, P., Evason-Coombe, C., Edmonds, M., Heckstall-Smith, E.M., Fleming, P. (2009). Hazardous cosleeping environments and risk factors amenable to change: case-control study of SIDS in south west England. *BMJ, 339,* b3666.

56. Carpenter, R., McGarvey, C., Mitchell, E.A., et al. (2013). Bed sharing when parents do not smoke: is there a risk of SIDS? An individual level analysis of five major case–control studies. *BMJ Open, 3,* e002299. doi:10.1136/bmjopen-2012-002299

57. Blair, P.S., Sidebotham, P., Pease, A., & Fleming, P.J. (2014). Bed-sharing in the absence of hazardous circumstances: is there a risk of sudden infant death syndrome? An analysis from two case-control studies conducted in the UK. *PLoS One, 9(9),* e107799.

58. Blabey, M.H. & Gessner, B.D. (2009). Infant bed-sharing practices and associated risk factors among births and infant deaths in Alaska. *Public Health Rep, 124(4),* 527–534.

59. Lahr, M.B., Rosenberg, K.D., & Laipidus, J.A. (2005). Bedsharing and maternal smoking in a population-based survey of new mothers. *Pediatrics, 116(4),* e530-42.

60. Forste, R., Weiss, J., & Lippincott, E. (2001). The decision to breastfeed in the United States: does race matter? *Pediatrics, 108(2),* 291–6.

61. Chen, A. & Rogan, W. (2004). Breast feeding and the risk of post-neonatal death in the United States. *Pediatrics, 113,* e435–e439.

62. Doucleff, M. (2018). Is Sleeping With Your Baby As Dangerous As Doctors Say? *NPR.* Retrieved from www.npr.org/sections/goatsandsoda/2018/05/21/601289695/is-sleeping-with-your-baby-as-dangerous-as-doctors-say

63. Bombard, J.M., et al. (2018). Vital Signs: Trends and Disparities in Infant Safe Sleep Practices - United States, 2009–2015. *Morbidity and Mortality Weekly Report, 67(1),* 39–46. doi:10.15585/mmwr.mm6701e1

64. Mitchell, E.A., et al. (2016). The Recent Fall in Postperinatal Mortality in New Zealand and the Safe Sleep Programme. *Acta Paediatrica, 105(11),* 1312–1320. doi:10.1111/apa.13494

65. American Academy of Pediatrics. (2019). AAP Facts. Retrieved from https://www.aap.org/en-us/about-the-aap/aap-facts/Pages/AAP-Facts.aspx

66. Sheppard, J. (2015). Does Co Sleeping Lead to SIDS? What the AAP Doesn't Tell You. *Healthy Child.* Retrieved from www.healthychild.com/does-co-sleeping-lead-to-sids/

67. Colson, E.R., Willinger, M., Rybin, D., et al. (2013). Trends and factors associated with infant bed sharing, 1993–2010: The National Infant Sleep Position Study. *JAMA Pediatrics, 167(11),* 1032–1037. doi:10.1001/jamapediatrics.2013.2560

68. Sackett, D.L., et al. (1996). Evidence based medicine: what it is and what it isn't. *BMJ, 312,* 71.

69. Mencken, H.L. (1917). The Divine Afflatus. *New York Evening Mail.*

70. Institute of Medicine (U.S.) Committee on Quality of Health Care in America. (2001). *Crossing the Quality Chasm: A New Health System for the 21st Century.* Washington (D.C.): National Academies Press.

71. Winter, C. (1999, September 30). Parents' Bed Unsafe for Babies, Study Says. *South Florida Sun Sentinel.* Retrieved from https://www.sun-sentinel.com/

72. Nakamura, S., Wind, M., Danello, M.A. (1999). Review of hazards associated with children placed in adult beds. *Archives of Pediatrics and Adolescent Medicine,* 153(10), 1019–23.

73. International Chiropractic Pediatric Association. (2008). Sleeping with Your Infant: Looking at the Facts. Retrieved from icpa4kids.org/fr/Wellness-Research/sleeping-with-your-infant-looking-at-the-facts.html

74. Sokol, Marian. (2005, May 10). Babies belong in cribs [Letter to the editor]. *San Antonio Express-News, 6B.* Courtesy of the Express-News archives.

75. Lin, R.G. (2008, April 24). Infant deaths prompt warning. *Los Angeles Times.* Retrieved from https://www.latimes.com/

76. Milwaukee Health Department. (n.d.) Safe Sleep Campaign. Retrieved from city.milwaukee.gov/health/Safe-Sleep-Campaign#.XFIGAc9Ki52

77. Haskell, C. (2011). Anti-Co-Sleeping Campaign Went Too Far. *The Stir.* Retrieved from https://thestir.cafemom.com/

78. Kendall-Tackett, K. (2012). Don't Sleep with Big Knives: Interesting (and Promising) Developments in the Mother-Infant Sleep Debate. *Clinical Lactation, 3(1),* 9–12. Retrieved from uslca.org/clinical-lactation

79. CDC/NCHS. (2018). National Vital Statistics System, Compressed Mortality File. Retrieved from www.cdc.gov/sids/data.htm

80. Blair, P.S., Sidebotham, P., Berry, P.J., Evans, M., & Fleming, P.J. (2006b). Major epidemiological changes in sudden infant death syndrome: A 20-year population-based study. *Lancet, 367,* 314–319.

81. Illinois Department of Children and Family Services. (2018). The ABC's of Safe Sleep. Retrieved from https://www2.illinois.gov

82. Smith, L.J. (2014). Sleeping Like A Mammal: Nighttime Realities for Childbirth Educators to Share With Parents. *Connecting the Dots.* Retrieved from https://www.lamaze.org/

83. Moon, R.Y., Mathews, A., Joyner, B.L., Oden, R.P., He, J., & McCarter, R. (2017). Health Messaging and African-American Infant Sleep Location: A Randomized Controlled Trial. *Journal of Community Health, 42(1),* 1–9. doi:10.1007/s10900-016-0227-1

84. Caraballo, M., Shimasaki, S., Johnston, K., Tung, G., Albright, K., Halbower, A. (2016). Knowledge, attitudes and risk for sudden unexpected death in children of adolescent mothers: A qualitative Study. *Journal of Pediatrics.* doi:10.1016 2016.03.031

85. Pro, A.P. (2009). Family: Without the Family Bed? *Mothering Magazine,* 48-49e.

86. Reite, M. & Field, T.M. (1985). *The Psychobiology of Attachment and Separation.* NY: Academic Press.

87. Mosko, S., Richard, C., & McKenna, J.J. (1997a). Infant arousals during mother–infant bed sharing: Implications for infant sleep and sudden infant death syndrome research. *Pediatrics, 100,* 841–849.

88. Bergman, N. (n.d.) Skin-To-Skin Contact – Background. Retrieved from http://skin2skincontact.com/research/background/

89. Bowlby, J. (1959). Separation anxiety. *International Journal of Psycho-Analytics, XLI,* 1–25.

90. Rosenblith, J.F., & Anderson-Huntington, R.B. (1977). Defensive Reactions to Stimulation of the Nasal and Oral Regions in Newborns: Relations to state. *Development of Upper Respiratory Anatomy and Function: Implications for Sudden Infant Death Syndrome*, Publication (NIH), 75–941. J.F. Bosma and J. Showacre. (Eds.) Bethesda: Department of Health, Education, and Welfare.

91. Valdes-Dapena, M. (1967). Sudden and Unexpected Death in Infancy: A Review of the World Literature, 1954-1966. *Pediatrics, 39(1)*, 129.

92. Hofer, M.A. (1992). Early relationships as regulators of infant physiology and behavior. *Acta Paediatrica, Supplement 1(397)*, 9–18. doi: 10.1111/j.1651-2227.1994.tb13260.x

93. Thoman, E.B. & Graham, S.E. (1986). Self-regulation of stimulation by premature infants. *Pediatrics, 78*, 855–60.

94. Stewart, M.W. & Stewart, L.A. (1991). Modification of sleep respiratory patterns by auditory stimulation: indications of techniques for preventing sudden infant death syndrome. *Sleep, 14(3)*, 241–8.

95. Mosko, S., Richard, C., McKenna, J.J., Drummond, S., & Mukai, D. (1997). Maternal proximity and infant $CO_2$ environment during bedsharing and possible implications for SIDS research. *American Journal of Physical Anthropology, 103(3)*, 315–328.

96. Papousek, M. & von Hofacker, N. (1998). Persistent crying in early infancy: A non-trivial condition of risk for the developing mother-infant relationship. *Child: Care, Health and Development, 24*, 395–424. doi:10.1046/j.1365-2214.2002.00091.x

97. McKenna, J.J., Ball, H.L., & Gettler, L.T. (2007). Mother-infant co-sleeping, breastfeeding and sudden infant death syndrome: What biological anthropology has discovered about normal infant sleep and pediatric sleep medicine. *Yearbook of Physical Anthropology, 50*, 133–161.

98. McKenna, J.J. (2014). Night waking among breastfeeding mothers and infants: Conflict, congruence or both? *Evolution, Medicine, and Public Health*, 40–47. doi:10.1093/emph/eou006

99. Ball, H.L. (2006a). Parent-infant bed-sharing behavior: effects of feeding type, and presence of father. *Human Nature. 17(3)*, 301–18.

100. Gettler, L.T., et al. (2012). Does Cosleeping Contribute to Lower Testosterone Levels in Fathers? Evidence from the Philippines. *PLoS ONE, 7(9)*. doi:10.1371/journal.pone.0041559

101. Konner, M. & Worthman, C. (1980). Nursing frequency, gonadal function, and birth spacing among !Kung hunter-gatherers. *Science, 207*, 788–791.

102. Dewey, K.G. (1998). Growth characteristics of breast-fed compared to formula-fed infants. *Biology of the Neonate, 74*, 94–105.

103. Vennemann, M.M., Bajanowski, T., Jorch, G., & Mitchell, E.A. (2009). Does Breastfeeding Reduce the Risk of Sudden Infant Death Syndrome? *Pediatrics, 123(3)*, e406–e410.

104. American Academy of Pediatrics. (2005). Section on Breastfeeding. Policy Statement: Organizational Principles to Guide and Define the Child Health Care System and / or Improve the Health of All Children. Retrieved from https://pediatrics.aappublications.org

105. Ball, H.L. (2003). Breastfeeding, bed-sharing and infant sleep. *Birth, Issues in Prenatal Care, 30(3)*, 181–188.

106. Gettler, L.T. (2012). Direct male care and hominin evolution: why male-child interaction is more than a nice social idea. *American Anthropologist, 112(1)*, 7–21. doi:10.1111/j.1548-1433.2009.01193.x

107. Møller, A.P. (2013). The evolution of monogamy: Mating relationships, parental care and sexual selection. *Monogamy: Mating strategies and partnerships in birds, humans and other mammals*. UK: Cambridge University Press. 29–41. doi:10.1017/CBO9781139087247.002

108. Gettler, L.T., et al. (2011). Longitudinal evidence that fatherhood decreases testosterone in human males. *PNAS, 108(39)*, 16194–16199. doi:10.1073/pnas.1105403108

109. Gettler, L.T., Feranil, A., McDade, T.W., & Kuzawa, C.W. (2015). Longitudinal Perspectives on Fathers' Residence Status, Time Allocation, and Testosterone in the Philippines. *Adaptive Human Behavior and Physiology, 1(2)*, 124–149.

110. Gettler, L.T., Agustin, S.S., McDade, T.W., & Kuzawa, C.W. (2011b). Short-term changes in fathers' hormones during father-child play: Impacts of paternal attitudes and experience. *Hormones and Behavior, 60(11)*, 599–606.

111. Gettler, L.T. (2016). Testosterone, fatherhood, and social networks. Trevathan, W.R., Rosenberg, K.R. (Eds.) *Costly and Cute: How Helpless Newborns Made Us Human.* Santa Fe, NM: School for Advanced Research. 149–176.

112. Gettler, L.T., McDade, T.W., Feranil, A.B., & Kuzawa, C.W. (2012a). Prolactin, fatherhood, and reproductive behavior in human males. *American Journal of Physical Anthropology, 148(3)*, 362–370.

113. Gettler, L.T. (2014). Applying Socioendocrinology to Evolutionary Models: Fatherhood and Physiology. *Evolutionary Anthropology, 23(4)*, 146–160. doi: 10.1002/evan.21412

114. Leech, S. (2006). Parent Infant Sleep Synchrony: A Test of Two Infant Sleep Locations. Master's Thesis. Department of Anthropology, Durham University.

115. McKenna, J.J. (2000). Cultural influences on infant and childhood sleep biology and the science that studies it: Toward a more inclusive paradigm. *Sleep and Breathing In Children: A Developmental Approach.* J. Laughlin, C. Marcos, J. Carroll. (Eds.) NY: Marcel-Dekker Pub, 99–130.

116. McKenna, J.J. & McDade, T. (2005). Why babies should never sleep alone: a review of the co-sleeping controversy in relation to SIDS, bedsharing and breast feeding. *Paediatric Respiratory Reviews, 6(2)*, 134–152. doi:10.1016/j.prrv.2005.03.006

117. Lucas, A., Morley, R., et al. (1992). Breast milk and subsequent intelligence quotient in children born preterm. *The Lancet, 339*, 261–264.

118. Deoni, S.C., Dean, D.C., Piryatinsky, I., O'Muirecheart, J., & Waskiewiez, N. (2013). Breastfeeding and early white matter development: a cross sectional study. *Neuroimage, 82*, 77–86. doi:10.1016/j.neuroimage.2013.05.090

119. Mileva-Seitz, V.R., Bakermans-Kranenburg, M., Battaini, C., & Luijk, M. (2016). Parent-child bed-sharing: The good, the bad, and the burden of evidence. *Sleep Medicine Reviews, 32.* doi:10.1016/j.smrv.2016.03.003

120. Anderson, G.C. (1995). Touch and the kangaroo care method. *Touch in Early Development.* T.M. Field. (Ed.) NJ: Lawrence Erlbaum, 33–51.

121. Goldstein Ferber, S., & Makhoul, I.R. (2004). The Effect of Skin-to-Skin Contact (Kangaroo Care) Shortly After Birth on the Neurobehavioral Responses of the Term Newborn: A Randomized, Controlled Trial. *Pediatrics, 113(4).* doi:10.1542/peds.113.4.858

122. Boundy, E.O. (2016). Kangaroo Mother Care and Neonatal Outcomes: A Meta Analysis. *Pediatrics, 137(1).* doi: 10.1542/peds.2015-2238

123. Winberg, J. (2005). Mother and newborn baby: mutual regulation of physiology and behavior—a selective review. *Developmental Psychobiology, 47(3)*, 217–29. doi:10.1002/dev.20094

124. Ludington-Hoe, S.M., Nguyen, N., Swinth, J.Y., & Satyshur, R.D. (2000). Kangaroo Care Compared to Incubators in Maintaining Body Warmth in Preterm Infants. *Biological Research For Nursing, 2(1)*, 60–73.

125. Ludington-Hoe, S., et al. (1999). Birth-related fatigue in 34–36-week preterm neonates: rapid recovery with very early kangaroo (skin-to-skin) care. *Journal of Obstetric, Gynecologic, and Neonatal Nursing, 28(1)*, 94–103.

126. Wiberg, B. & de Chateau, P. (1977). Long-term effect on mother-infant behaviour of extra contact during the first hour post partum. II. A follow-up at three months. *Acta Paediatrica, 66(2)*, 145–151.

127. Rigda, R.S., et al. (2000). Bed sharing patterns in a cohort of Australian infants during the first six months after birth. *Journal of Pediatrics and Child Health, 36(2)*, 117–121.

128. Widstrom, A., et al. (1990). Short term effects of early suckling and touch of the nipple on maternal behaviour. *Early Human Development, 21*, 153–163.

129. Vial-Courmont, M. (2000). The kangaroo ward. *Med Wieku Rozwoj, 4(2 suppl 3)*, 105–117.

130. Brazy, J.E. (1988). Effects of crying on cerebral blood volume and cytochrome aa3. *The Journal of Pediatrics, 112*, 457–461.

131. Australian Association for Infant Mental Health. (2002). Controlled Crying. *Position Paper 1.*

132. Elias, M.F., Nicholson, N., Bora, C., & Johnston, J. (1986). Sleep-wake patterns of breast-fed infants in the first two years of life. *Pediatrics 77(3)*, 322–329.

133. Elias, M.F., Nicholson, N.A., & Konner, M. (1986). Two sub-cultures of maternal care in the United States. *Current perspectives in primate social dynamics*. D. M. Taub and F. A. King (Eds.) NY: Van Nostrand Reinhold. 37–50.

134. University of British Columbia. (2017). Holding infants—or not—can leave traces on their genes: Amount of close and comforting contact from caregivers changes children's molecular profile. *ScienceDaily*. Retrieved from www.sciencedaily.com/releases/2017/11/171127094928.htm

135. Moore, S.R., McEwen, L.M., Quirt, J., Morin, A., Mah, S.M., Barr, R.G.,...& Kobor, M.S. (2017). Epigenetic correlates of neonatal contact in humans. *Development and Psychopathology, 29(05)*, 1517. doi:10.1017/S0954579417001213

136. Nield, D. (2019). Babies Who Get Cuddled More Seem to Have Their Genetics Changed For Years Afterwards. *ScienceAlert*. Retrieved from www.sciencealert.com/cuddling-babies-alters-genetics-dna-for-years

137. McKenna, J.J., Middlemiss, W., & Tarsha, M. (2016). Potential Evolutionary, Neurophysiological, and Developmental Origins of Sudden Infant Death Syndrome and Inconsolable Crying (Colic): Is It About Controlling Breath? *Family Relations, 65*, 239–258. doi:10.1111/fare.12178

138. Hunziker, U.A. & Barr, R.G. (1986). Increased Carrying Reduces Infant Crying: A Randomized Controlled Trial. *Pediatrics, 77(5)*.

139. Barr, R.G., Kenner, M., Bakeman, R., & Adamson, L. (1991). Crying in !Kung San Infants: A Test of the Cultural Specificity Hypothesis. *Developmental Medicine and Child Neurology, 33*, 601–610.

140. Poets, Christian. (2004). Apparent life-threatening events and the sudden infant death on a monitor. *Paediatric Respiratory Reviews, 5 (Suppl 1)*, S383–S386.

141. Meny, R.G., Carroll, J.L., Carbone, M.T., Kelly, D.H. (1994). Cardiorespiratory Recordings from infants dying suddenly and unexpectedly at home. *Pediatrics, 92(1)*, 43–49.

142. Fleming, P.J., Levine, M.R., Azaz, Y., Wigfield, R., & Steward, A.J. (1993). Interactions between thermoregulation and the control of respiration in infants: Possible relationship to sudden infant death. *Acta Paediatrica, 82 (Suppl 389)*, 57–59.

143. Fleming, P.J., Howell, T., Wigfield, R., et al. (1994). The effects of thermal care, maternal smoking and breastfeeding on respiratory illness in infants. *Pediatric Pulmonology, 18*, 391.

144. Fleming, P.J., Young, J., & Blair, P.S. (2006). The importance of mother-baby interactions in determining nighttime thermal conditions for sleeping infants: Observations from the home and the sleep laboratory. *Paediatric Child Health, 11 (Suppl A)*, 7A–10A.

145. Tsogt, B., Manaseki-Holland, S., Pollock, J., Blair, P.S., & Fleming, P.J. (2016). Thermoregulatory effects of swaddling in Mongolia: a randomised controlled study. *Archives of Disease in Childhood, 101(2)*, 152–160.

146. National Sleep Foundation. (2005). Sleep in America Poll. Retrieved from www.sleepfoundation.org/_content/hottopics/2005 _summary_of_findings.pdf

147. Newcombe, P.A., et al. (1994). Lactation and reduced risk of premenopausal breast cancer. *New England Journal of Medicine, 330(2)*, 81–87.

148. Ainsworth, M.D.S., Blehar, M.C., Waters, E., & Wall, S. (1978). *Patterns of attachment: A psychological study of the strange situation*. UK: Lawrence Erlbaum.

149. Bartick, M., Steube, A., Schwarz, E.B., Bimla, E., Luongo, C., Reinhold, A., et al. (2013). Cost analysis of maternal disease associated with suboptimal breastfeeding. *Obstetrics & Gynecology, 122(1)*, 111–9. doi:10.1097/AOG.0b013e318297a047

150. Somers, R.L. (2012). Assessment of infant mattress firmness: a do-it-yourself safety test to reduce the risk of asphyxiation. *Australian and New Zealand Journal of Public Health, 36(5)*, 490–491. doi:10.1111/j.1753-6405.2012.00920.x

151. Fleming, P., Blair, P., Bacon, C., et al. (1996). Environments of infants during sleep and the risk of the sudden infant death syndrome: Results of 1993–1995 case control study for confidential inquiry into stillbirths and deaths in infancy. *British Medical Journal, 313*, 191–195.

152. Bertrand, K.A., Hanan, N.J., Honerkamp-Smith, G., Best, B.M., & Chambers, C.D. (2018). Marijuana Use by Breastfeeding Mothers and Cannabinoid Concentrations in Breast Milk. *Pediatrics, 142(3)*. doi:10.1542/peds.2018-1076

153. Rainey, M. (2016). Coroner's warning over cannabis use and co-sleeping after baby death. *News Letter*.

154. Tinsworth, D. K., and McDonald, J. E. (2002). Hazard Analysis: Crib-Related Deaths. Retrieved from https://cpsc.gov

155. Carroll-Pankhurst, C. & Mortimer, A. (2001). Sudden infant death syndrome, bed-sharing, parental weight, and age at death. *Pediatrics, 107(3)*, 530–536.

156. Gettler, L.T. & McKenna, J.J. (2010). Never Sleep with Baby? Or Keep Me Close But Keep Me Safe: Eliminating Inappropriate 'Safe Infant Sleep' Rhetoric in the United States. *Current Pediatric Reviews, 6(1)*, 71–77. doi:10.2174/157339610791317250

157. Bergman, A.M. (2013). Bedsharing per se Is Not Dangerous. *Journal of the American Medical Association (JAMA) Pediatrics, 167(11)*, 998–999. doi:10.1001/jamapediatrics.2013.2569

158. Gromada-Kerkoff, K. (1985). *Mothering Multiples: Breast Feeding and Caring For Twins*. IL: La Leche League International. (3rd Rev. ed. 2007).

159. Lutes, L.M. & Altimer, L. (2001). Co-bedding multiples. *Newborn and nursing reviews, 1(4)*. Retrieved from www.nainr.com/scripts /om.dll/serv

160. Nyqvist, K.H. & Lutes, L.M. (1998). Co-bedding twins: a developmentally supportive care strategy. *Journal of Obstetrical, Gynecological, and Neonatal Nursing, 27(4)*, 450–56.

161. Ball, H.L. (2006). Caring for twins: sleeping arrangements and their implications. *Evidence Based Midwifery, 4(1)*, 10–16.

162. Ball, H.L. (2008). Together or Apart? A behavioral and physiological investigation of sleeping arrangements for twin babies. *Midwifery in press. 23(4)*, 404–12. doi:10.1016/j.midw.2006.07.004

163. Dawkins, C.R. (1976) *The Selfish Gene*. UK: Oxford University Press.

164. Pennestri, M.H., et al. (2018). Uninterrupted infant sleep, Development, and Maternal Mood. *Pediatrics, 142*, e20174330.

165. Middlemiss, W., Granger, D.A., Goldberg, W.A., & Nathans, L.A. (2012). Asynchrony of mother-infant hypothalamic-pituitary-adrenal axis activity following extinction of infant crying responses induced during the transition to sleep. *Early Human Development, 88*, 227–232.

166. Douglas, P.S., & Hill, P.S. (2013). Behavioral sleep interventions in the first six months of life do not improve outcomes for mothers or infants: a systematic review. *The Journal of Developmental and Behavioral Pediatrics, 34*, 497–507. doi:10.1097/DBP.0b013e31829cafa6

167. Konner, M. (2010). *The Evolution of Childhood: Relationships, Emotion, Mind*. UK: The Belknap Press of Harvard University Press.

168. Pease, A.S., et al. (2016). "Swaddling and the Risk of Sudden Infant Death Syndrome: A Meta-analysis." *Pediatrics, 137(6)*.

169. McKenna J.J., & Gettler, L.T. (2008). Cultural influences on infant sleep biology and the science that studies it: toward a more inclusive paradigm, part II. *In Sleep and Breathing In Children: A Developmental Approach, 2*, 183–221. G. Loughlin, J. Carroll and C. Marcus (Eds). NY: Marcel Dekker.

170. Forbes, J.F., Weiss, D.S., & Folen, R.A. (1992). The Cosleeping Habits of Military Children. *Military Medicine, 157(4)*, 196–200. doi:10.1093/milmed/157.4.196

171. Crawford, C.J. (1994). Parenting practices in the Basque country: Implications of infant and childhood sleeping location for personality development. *Ethos, 22(1)*, 42–82. doi.org/10.1525/eth.1994.22.1.02a00020

172. Germo, G.R., Chang, E.S., Keller, M.A., & Goldberg, W.A. (2007). Child sleep arrangements and family life: perspectives from mothers and fathers. *Infant and Child Development, 16*, 433–456. doi.org/10.1002/icd

173. Germo, G.R., Goldberg, W.A., & Keller, M.A. (2009). Learning to sleep through the night: solution or strain for mothers and young children? *Infant Mental Health Journal, 30*, 223e44. doi.org/10.1002/imhj

174. Okami, P., Wesiner, T., & Olmstead, R. (2004). Outcome Correlates of Parent-Child Bedsharing: An Eighteen-Year Longitudinal Study. *Journal of Developmental & Behavioral Pediatrics, 23*, 244–253. doi:10.1097/00004703-200208000-00009

175. Mosenkis, J. (1998). The Effects of Childhood Cosleeping On Later Life Development. Master's Thesis. University of Chicago. Chicago, IL.

176. Keller, M., & Goldberg, W. (2004). Co-sleeping: Help or hindrance for young children's independence? *Infant and Child Development, 13(5)*, 369–388. doi:10.1002/icd.365

177. Heron, P. (1994). Non-Reactive Cosleeping and Child Behavior: Getting a Good Night's Sleep All Night, Every Night. Master's thesis. Department of Psychology, University of Bristol.

178. Lewis, R.J. & Janda, L.H. (1998). The Relationship between Adult Sexual Adjustment and Childhood Experience regarding Exposure to Nudity, Sleeping in the Parental Bed, and Parental Attitudes toward Sexuality. *Archives of Sexual Behavior, 17*, 349–363.

179. Javo, C., Rønning, J.A., Heyerdahl, S., & Rudmin, F.W. (2004). Parenting correlates of child behavior problems in a multiethnic community sample of preschool children in northern Norway. *European Child & Adolescent Psychiatry, 13(1)*, 8–18.

180. Holmes, J. (1993). *John Bowlby and Attachment Theory*. UK: Taylor & Francis, Inc. 181.

181. Teti, D.M., Crosby, B., McDaniel, B.T., Shimizu, M., & Whitesell, C.J. (2015). Marital and emotional adjustment in mothers and infant sleep arrangements during the first six months. *Monographs of the Society for Research in Child Development, 80*, 160e76. doi.org/10.1111/mono.12150

182. Crowell, J., Keener, M., Ginsburg, N., & Anders, T. (1987). Sleep habits in toddlers 18 to 36 months old. *Journal of the American Academy of Child and Adolescent Psychiatry, 26*, 510e5.

183. Wailoo, M., Ball, H.L., Fleming, P.J., & Ward-Platt, M.P. (2004). Infants bed-sharing with mothers: helpful, harmful or don't we know? *Archives of Disease in Childhood, 89(12)*, 1082–1083. doi:10.1136/adc.2004.054312

184. American Academy of Pediatrics Policy Statement. (2016). SIDS and Other Sleep-Related Infant Deaths: Updated 2016 Recommendations for a Safe Infant Sleeping Environment. *Pediatrics, 138(5)*.

185. Blair, P.S. (2008). Putting co-sleeping into perspective. *Jornal de Pediatria, 84(2)*, 99–101. doi:10.1590/S0021-75572008000200001

186. Ball, H.L., Tomori, C., McKenna, J.J. (2019). Toward an Integrated Anthropology of Infant Sleep. *American Anthropologist*. doi:10.1111/aman.13284

187. Kennedy, J.F. (1962). Yale University Commencement.

188. McKenna, J. (1996). Sudden Infant Death Syndrome in Cross-Cultural Perspective: Is Infant-Parent Cosleeping Protective? *Annual Review of Anthropology, 25(1)*, 201–216. doi:10.1146/annurev.anthro.25.1.201

189. Bartick, M., & Tomori, C. (2018). Sudden infant death and social justice: A syndemics approach. *Maternal & Child Nutrition*, e12652. http://doi.org/10.1111/mcn.12652

190. Blair, P.S., Ball, H., McKenna, J.J., Winter, L., Marinelli, K., & Bartick, M. (2019). Bedsharing and Breastfeeding. *Academy of Breastfeeding Medicine Protocol #6, revision*.

191. Bartick, M., & Smith, L.J. (2014). Speaking Out on Safe Sleep: Evidence-Based Infant Sleep Recommendations. *Breastfeeding Medicine:* The official journal of the Academy of Breastfeeding Medicine. doi:9.10.1089/bfm.2014.0113

# APPENDIX VIII
# Index